Home Health Outcomes and Resource Utilization:
Integrating Today's Critical Priorities

Carolyn E. Adams, EdD, RN, CNAA
and Ann L. Anthony, MS, RN
Editors

National League for Nursing
New York
Pub. No. 19-7246

Copyright (c) 1997
National League for Nursing
350 Hudson Street, New York, NY 10014

All rights reserved. No part of this book may be reproduced in print, or by photostatic means, or in any other manner, without the express written permission of the publisher.

ISBN 0-88737-724-6

> The views expressed in this publication represent the views of the authors and do not necessarily reflect the official views of the National League for Nursing.

This book was copy edited by Linda Greer.
Graphic Design by George Gerard Design. Typography by Dan Diggles.

Printed in the United States of America

We want to thank our colleagues at the National League for Nursing for their support and encouragement with this monograph series. We would like to especially express our appreciation to Dr. Lynda Crawford, Associate Director for the Center for Research in Nursing Education and Community Health, for her energy and continued attention to the many details involved in the project. A special thanks goes to Dr. Delroy Louden, Executive Director for Research in Nursing Education and Community Health, for his inspiration and mentoring.

Carolyn E. Adams
Ann L. Anthony

EDITORIAL REVIEW BOARD

Editors

Carolyn E. Adams, EdD, RN, CNAA
Associate Professor
Intercollegiate Center for Nursing Education
Washington State University

Ann L. Anthony, MS, RN
Director, Program Development
Connecticut Association for Home Care, and
President, Anthony and Associates
Consultants in Home Health Care Management

Editorial Review Board

Nancy Biggerstaff, MN, RN
Care Resources Coordinator
Group Health Northwest
Spokane, Washington

Jayne Furness Moore, PhD, RN
Case Manager
Family Home Care
Spokane, Washington

Judith Hriceniak, PhD, RN
Chairperson/Professor
Central Connecticut State University
New Britain, Connecticut

Valdyne M. Viers, PhD, RN, CNS
Research Associate
Scott & White Health Care System
Temple, Texas

Carolyn J. Humphrey, MS, RN
Editor
Home Healthcare Nurse
Louisville, Kentucky

CONTRIBUTING AUTHORS

Carolyn E. Adams, EdD, RN, CNAA
Associate Professor
Intercollegiate Center for Nursing Education
Washington State University

Theresa S. Ayer, MS, RN, CNAA
President and COO
Community Health Accreditation Program, Inc.

Barbara Boyd, BSN, RN
Administrator
Home and Community Services
Department of Community Health and Long Term Care
Group Health Cooperative of Puget Sound

Susan Brink, BSN, RN
Candidate, Masters of Science in Nursing
Nursing Management and Policy Program
Yale University School of Nursing

Cynthia Drucker, BSN, CPHQ
Quality Improvement Manager
Visiting Nurse Services of the Northwest
Everett, WA

Jan Herzog, MSN, RN
Clinical Program Development Analyst
Visiting Nurse Association of Greater Philadelphia

Julu Huang, BSN, RN
Candidate, Masters of Science in Nursing
Nursing Management and Pollicy Program
Yale University School of Nursing

Karen Levine, BSN, RN
Candidate, Masters of Science in Nursing
Nursing Management and Pollicy Program
Yale University School of Nursing

Mary P. Malone, MS, JD, CHE
Vice President, Corporate Development
Press, Ganey Associates, Inc

Paula Milone-Nuzzo, PhD, RN
Associate Professor and Chair
Specialty Care and Managment Division
Yale University School of Nursing

Nancy Moran, MS, RN
Press, Ganey Associates, Inc

Moira O'Neill, BSN, RN
Candidate, Masters of Science in Nursing
Nursing Management and Pollicy Program
Yale University School of Nursing
Division of International Health
Yale University School of Public Health

Joanne Ozaki-Moore, BSN, MEd
Patient Services Manager
Visiting Nurse Services of the Northwest
Everett, WA

Karen Pace, MSN, RN
Vice President
Research, Regulatory Affairs and Education
National Association for Home Care

Mary Ann Popovich
Director, Home Care Division
Joint Commission on Accreditation of Healthcare Organizations

Joanne Rokosky, MSN
Clinical and Staff Development Specialist
Visiting Nurse Services of the Northwest
Everett, WA

Bernard Rose
Business Manager
Community Health Accreditation Program, Inc.

Mary Schoen, MSN, MPH, RN
Director of Education Services
Visiting Nurse Association of Greater Philadelphia

Robert Short, PhD
Research Associate
Washington State University
Spokane, WA

PREFACE

NLN's Center for Research in Nursing Education and Community Health monograph series is designed to enable nurses and other health care professionals to explore current issues around education, practice and research in a timely fashion. Cutting edge articles are peer- reviewed with dispatch to reflect the rapid changes in the health care environment. The series addresses the broad range of issues relevant to nurse educators dealing with the changing landscape of nursing in terms of both education and policy.

Delroy Louden
Lynda Crawford
Donna Post

INTRODUCTION TO MONOGRAPH SERIES

Home Health Outcomes and Resource Utilization: Integrating Today's Critical Priorities

Today, we live and work in one of the most exciting and challenging periods in the evolution of health care in America. We have seen more change in the past decade than we have during the past century. More than ever before, health care has come "home" . . . to the patient's home and to the patient's community. How well we plan for this care will determine the "shape" of America's health care for its people.

The Council of Community Health Services of the National League for Nursing is pleased to play a pivotal role in this process by introducing this monograph series for students, faculty, and practitioners in community-health nursing. The purpose of the Council of Community Health Series is to provide leadership in matters related to nursing and in the delivery of quality health care by community-health agencies and to assist agencies in the development and improvement of their service programs. Council membership includes a broad representation from the fields of nursing education, home health care, and public health.

A monograph is a collection of writings which address a single subject, from a variety of perspectives, within one publication. A monograph series was selected as the best format so the reader will be able to access quickly the most relevant and contemporary thoughts and dynamic information available on a specific topic. Health care is in the midst of incredible and accelerated change. It is becoming extremely difficult for students, educators, and providers to remain current in their knowledge of contemporary community-health issues. This monograph series will assist the reader to locate the best resources on selected topics within one publication, without conducting individual, time-consuming literature searches.

Each year a new volume of the series will be published by the Council of Community Health Services as a benefit to those interested in community-based practice and issues.

Ann Anthony
Co-Editor
Chairperson, Council for Community Health Services

INTRODUCTION TO VOLUME I

Home Health Outcomes and Resource Utilization: Integrating Today's Critical Resources

The overriding challenge in home health care is to balance quality patient outcomes with the resources used to attain them. Home-health administrators rate a reputation for delivering quality care as the most important success factor for a home-health agency. But quality patient outcomes are resource intensive, and, consequently, costly. The high cost of securing quality patient outcomes is occurring in a home-health environment where both public and private payers are determined to stabilize or reduce home-health costs. Home-health providers must identify mechanisms to enhance patient outcomes while maximizing resources.

In this monograph, the quality/resource-utilization equation in home health is examined from various perspectives, including that of home-health agency providers, accreditors, researchers, managed-care organizations, and the National Association of Home Care. Current strategies used by home-health agencies to enhance patient outcomes within constraints of shrinking revenues are described. Future industry standards are outlined, along with implications for quality and resource utilization.

Home-Health Outcomes and Resource Utilization: Integrating Today's Critical Resources is a valuable resource for home-health providers, nursing faculty, and students. Providers can obtain examples of tested methods for enhancing quality while conserving resources. Providers will find new information on home-health accreditation in the articles from the Joint Commission and the Community Health Accreditation Program (CHAP). The article on prospective payment heralds the payment mechanism for most home-health services in the future.

For faculty and students, the monograph provides in-depth, topical information. Home health is the fastest growing segment of the health-care industry, and many graduating students will practice in this field. Faculty can use the monograph to acquaint students with two of the most important areas in home health: quality and resource utilization. The agency-based articles can also be analyzed as management case studies; students can be guided to apply critical thinking techniques to the narrated processes and outcomes.

Carolyn E. Adams
Co-Editor

Contents

Contributing Authors   v
Preface   vii
Introduction to Monograph Series   viii
Introduction to Volume I   ix
Contents   x

1. **Measurement of Outcomes in Home Care: An Overview**   1
    by Paula Milone-Nuzzo, Susan Brink, Julu Huang, Karen Levine, and Moira O'Neill

2. **Outcome Data Analysis: Putting Results Into Practice**   21
    by Jan Herzog and Mary Schoen

3. **Critical Pathways Define Best Practice**   35
    by Joanne M. Rokosky, Cynthia Drucker, and Joanne Ozaki-Moore

4. **Registered Nurse Use and Patient Outcomes in Home Health**   51
    by Carolyn E. Adams and Robert Short

5. **Utilizing Patient Satisfaction to Meet the Challenges of Managed Health Care**   63
    by Nancy Yezzi Moran and Mary P. Malone

6. **Home-Health Quality and Resource Utilization in a Managed-Care Organization**   79
    by Barbara Boyd

7. Initiatives Aim to Integrate Performance
    Measures Into the Joint Commission's
    Accreditation Process   89
    by Maryanne Popovich

8. The Chap Benchmarking Program:
    A Systematic Measurement of Outcomes
    to Enhance Resource Utilization   97
    by Theresa S. Ayer and Bernard Rose

9. Prospective Payment: Impact on
    Resource Utilization and Quality   109
    by Karen Beckman Pace

Chapter One

MEASUREMENT OF OUTCOMES IN HOME CARE: AN OVERVIEW

by Paula Milone-Nuzzo, RN, PhD, Associate Professor and Chair,
  Specialty Care and Management Division, Yale School of Nursing

Susan Brink, RN, BSN, Candidate, MS Nursing
Julu Huang, RN, BSN, Candidate, MS Nursing
Karen Levine, RN, BSN, Candidate, MS Nursing
Moira O'Neill, RN, BSN, Candidate, MS Nursing and Public Health
Nursing Management and Policy Program, Yale School of Nursing
Division of International Health, Yale University School of Public Health

Abstract

The measurement of outcomes in home care is essential to document changes in the patient's behaviors and health status. In addition, outcome measurement will provide the necessary data to demonstrate the impact of care provided in the home. Yet home care is struggling to operationally define outcome measurement and implement a uniform system to collect outcome data. This paper begins by describing the impact of the changing health-care delivery system on the home-care market. Selected models of outcome measurement are described, followed by a comparison of the data elements included in the outcomes-measurement system.

Introduction

Changes in the health-care delivery system have mandated that we pay increased attention to quality and the outcomes of care. Many home-care agencies are changing the way they view the measurement of outcomes as a result of increased competition, declining resources, and increasing accountability for the services they provide. Agencies are receiving the message from patients, physicians, and payers that outcomes measurement, as a vehicle for assessing quality of care, is critical to their long-term viability. The reputation of a home-care agency for providing quality care is critical to the success of that agency, since referrals and contracts are often based on documented quality the agency provides.[1]

"Outcomes" are defined as the measured changes in the patient's behavior between two points in time. Outcomes are the changes in patients that are measured in a systematic way between two or more points in time along the continuum of care.[2] Home-care providers are challenged to provide an accurate assessment of the patient and establish measurable goals, so that changes in the patient's behavior and health status can be documented.

Quality of care is another concept that is ubiquitous in many discussions about health-care delivery. "Quality" is defined as the degree to which patient care increases the likelihood of desirable outcomes and reduces the likelihood of undesirable outcomes.[3] Home-care agencies are required to maintain quality and measure outcomes, yet the myriad definitions, programs, and products to assess quality outcomes make these requirements difficult to implement.

Patients have long been interested in the quality of care provided by home-care agencies. As competition among home-care agencies and managed-care organizations increases, consumers are being encouraged to play an active role in deciding who will be their insurance company or home-care provider. One measure that consumers can use to assess the quality of the care provided by a home-care agency is the outcomes achieved by the patients.

Payers are particularly interested in measuring the outcomes of care. From a managed-care perspective, outcomes must consider the cost effectiveness and cost efficiency of the services provided in relationship to the measured changes in the patient's behavior and health status. Managed-care organizations are interested in identifying those agencies that demonstrate the most significant changes in the patient's behavior in a cost-effective manner. A home-health agency can use quality outcome information to publicize its strengths to the community, and attract referrals and contracts from managed-care organizations.

Physicians and other primary care providers are also interested in home-care outcomes. It is widely recognized that the goals of home care are not well understood by the physician community.[4–6] By articulating the measured changes in the patient's behavior after a home-care interaction, physicians and others will be able to view the tangible benefits of home health-care delivery.

There have been numerous attempts to measure the quality of care provided to patients in the home. The purpose of this manuscript is to explore the issues inherent in the current health-care delivery system that affect how outcomes are measured and quality is assured in home care. Selected outcomes measures will be described with a focus on OASIS (Outcomes Assessment and Information Set) as a system of outcome-information collection. Finally, a comparison of the data elements included in the outcome-measurement systems discussed will be presented.

Issues Affecting Home-Care Outcomes
Managed Care
Managed care is dramatically changing health-care delivery in the United States. There are numerous definitions of managed care, both in the literature and in practice. For the purposes of this discussion, managed care is defined as "a comprehensive approach to health-care delivery that encompasses planning and coordination of care, patient and provider education, monitoring of care quality and cost control."[7] Essential components of a managed-care plan include, but are not limited to, the management of access, cost, and the quality of health services.

The move to managed care has been pervasive in the private sector. Eckom[8] reported that 65% of workers in medium and large companies are now enrolled in some form of managed care. Blue Cross/Blue Shield has predicted that 90% of their membership will be in a managed plan by the year 2000. The American Managed Care and Review Association suggests that over 41% of the total population is now covered by managed-care organizations.[7] Like all other constituents of the health-care industry, home health-care providers struggle to respond to this change in reimbursement method and to predict both the effects and expectations of a managed-care structure. Fazzi and Agoglia conducted a national study of 50 managed-care organizations (MCOs) that revealed anticipated increases in home-care usage in the next two years. Three specific issues were of critical concern among these surveyed MCOs: clinical outcomes, patient satisfaction, and cost effectiveness. Cost-competitive services ranked extremely high among all the MCOs. Quality appeared to be equally important, with 90% stating that high-quality services are very important or required.[9] Clearly, cost cannot be addressed without also considering quality in the pursuit of desired clinical outcomes.

The challenge emerges when creating a comprehensive outcome measure to accurately track the three issues identified as important to MCOs and other third-party payers. An analysis of the responses to Fazzi and Agoglia's survey makes it clear that a home-care database should include data elements that are indicators of quality of services, cost effectiveness, and patient satisfaction.

Prospective Payment
A "prospective payment system" (PPS) is defined as a method of reimbursement that involves setting a rate for a specific amount of service before the service is provided. In a PPS, the ability to adjust for case mix is essential to the survival of the agency. The home-health agency must have the opportunity to adjust for case mix so they are not penalized for caring for a more complex population than the group upon which the predetermined payment was based.

PPS contains advantages and disadvantages for the home-care industry. The current cost-based, retroactive reimbursement system allows for payment adjustments as late as three years after interim payment is made. Under PPS, an agency will know in advance what payment it can expect. Agency budgets will be developed based on the projected revenues and care needs of the patients.

When managed-care organizations were asked to predict how they will reimburse home-care agencies, 50% foresaw a capitated approach that involves a prospective payment system.[9] In PPS, a dollar amount per condition or episode will replace number of visits. It will be the agency's responsibility to determine the most efficient way to care for the patient, given the resources available. This would be an advantage if the agencies are able to accurately predict the needs of the patients. If predictions are accurate, the home-care agency will be able to meet the patient's care needs within the payment provided, and perhaps even realize a small margin for the agency. If predictions are inaccurate, care needs will persist without reimbursement, and returns for the agency diminish.

This requires a change in thinking for the home-care industry. What will be needed at the agency level is an understanding of what resources are required to achieve specific clinical outcomes. At present, available home-care data include billing information and some inconsistent clinical data. The inconsistencies arise from the many different methods for collecting data in home-care agencies.

In 1996, a proposal for a Prospective Payment System (PPS) for Medicare Home Health Services was submitted to Congress. This plan was submitted as a more efficient alternative to other budget-reduction measures, including bundling of home-care payments with hospital payments and increasing co-payments.[10] By taking an active stance on the issue of prospective payments, home-care providers can maintain a voice in the unavoidable changes to the reimbursement structure.

The achievement of a successful PPS cannot be reached without a commitment to the collection of pertinent data in the industry. In recognizing the implications of a PPS, it is essential that all members of the home health-care industry acknowledge the importance of data collection to facilitate that process. Prospective pay can be an efficient and cost-effective system of reimbursement, but only if it is based on accurate and reliable data describing home health-care recipients and their needs.

Cost

There are many forces involved in the restructuring of the health-care payment system. Health-care spending in the United States continues to outpace the general national economy. Home care, the fastest growing component of the health-care industry, reflects the growing needs of an aging population and the increasing availability of sophisticated medical technologies in the home.[10] The Medicare hospital prospective payment system, instituted in 1984, initiated a trend toward shorter hospital stays, resulting in increased utilization of home care for many patients who traditionally would have remained in the hospital during recuperation.[11]

The growth of the home-care industry is reflected in the growth of home-care expenditures. Home health-care spending increased 583% between 1980 and 1991.[12] Medicare, as the largest single payer of home-care services, has become the fourth largest expense in the federal budget.[13] Regardless of whether the rise in expenditures represents merely a shift in spending, or a contributing factor in actual saving in the overall cost of health care, policy makers have taken note of this dramatic increase. Policy makers influencing Medicare expenditures are expected to demand a decrease in spending. Additionally, insurance companies and managed-care organizations will aggressively seek ways to cut or avoid costs.

Cost savings cannot be achieved arbitrarily. A strategic approach must be based on an analysis of patient characteristics, agency interventions, and resource use. The development of outcomes-based databases will provide the foundation for this analysis. Accurate outcome data is also necessary for the home-care agency to validate the effect of their interventions.

Predictors for Analysis
Our primary reason for providing health care is to benefit patients. In the context of analyzing issues about reimbursement, utilization, cost, and even political topics, it is possible for us to overlook the basic fact that the raison d'etre of health care is to influence patient outcomes.[14]

As early as 1850, Florence Nightingale recognized the value of predictive data. In 1859, she embarked on a campaign for the collection of uniform data to allow for comparisons of hospitals in different districts of the same county on variables such as mortality, case mix, and socioeconomic status of the patient.[15] Building on the early work of Nightingale, contemporary health-policy makers suggest it would be clinically and financially beneficial to develop and utilize data as predictors of need, resource use, and outcomes. Patient records are rich sources for review of the flow of practice. A database that includes uniform, precise, and concise documentation allows us to identify the worth and value of specific interventions.

One of the purposes of home care is to prevent patients from hospital or institutional readmission. Therefore, the use of predictors of readmission to hospital as part of a needs assessment for home care should identify those at greatest risk, and allow for appropriate supportive measures. Prescott, Soeken & Griggs concluded that the variables of diagnosis, age, initial length of stay, and prior use of hospital or emergency-room resources were significant predictors of hospital readmission. The significance of these variables increased when clinical and social factors were added to diagnostic and demographic information.[16]

Psychosocial and environmental indicators play a significant role in the clinical outcomes of home-care patients. Given that care is provided in the patient's home for a very brief period of time, all the variables that can have a deleterious effect on patients are unable to be controlled. For example, the effect of low income, poor sanitation, and community violence is negated by the controlled environment of the hospital. Home-care providers may not be able to address and correct all the psychological and environmental variables that affect health care, but these factors must be assessed on admission and integrated into the plan of care whenever possible, since they affect the quality, cost, and health outcomes that an agency and payer can expect to achieve.[17]

That variables are predictive of future trends underlies much scientific research. A great deal of nursing research seeks to identify and predict self-care deficits or changes in behavior. Such research provides a means for health-care providers to predict resource use, cost, patient needs, and patient satisfaction with a given service or intervention. If variables can be defined to make predictions about the need for home care, then a very rich and useful database could be developed.

Patient Satisfaction
Patient satisfaction, or customer satisfaction, is an integral component of outcomes measurement. "Patient satisfaction" is the extent to which a consumer is satisfied with the quality of the services provided by the provider. Studies have examined the extent to which a patient can assess the quality, including clinical quality, of the home-care experience. Many home-care patients are able to articulate what quality is, what their care is, and what they expect from the home-care episode.[18] Satisfaction is a critical quality indicator, and third-party payers are becoming increasingly interested in the results of satisfaction surveys. Decisions to utilize agencies may be based on performance records as perceived by the patient. In an increasingly competitive market, monitoring patient-satisfaction data may impact on an agency's market share and general level of success.

Home-care agencies have traditionally used agency-specific patient-satisfaction instruments to assess this aspect of patient outcome. Agencies developed instruments that included general questions about the services they provided. For example, they asked, "Are you satisfied with the care you have received from our agency?" The responses to this question provided little clarity for the quality-improvement efforts of the agency. Agency-developed patient-satisfaction instruments came as a result of the mandate to collect patient-satisfaction information and the lack of any standardized instruments that were relevant to home care.

Patient-satisfaction instruments have characteristically lacked the reliability and validity information that would allow for confidence in the data collected. Does a positive response to a question about satisfaction really mean the patient is satisfied with his/her care, or does it mean something else based on the phrasing of the question? Would the patient give the same responses to the survey two weeks from now as he gave today? In addition, since agencies tend to develop their own instrument, there is little similarity between individual questions that would allow for comparison of information across a state or region.

Standardized instruments for the collection of patient-satisfaction data have been developed and are currently being used in home care. These instruments are often equipped with norms or a standard by which individual home-care agencies can compare their results with other home-care agencies. MCOs are interested in patient satisfaction that can be compared across agencies and with specific populations. Standardized instruments allow for that comparison to occur. The main areas that are included in these instruments are availability, access, technical adequacy, sensitivity, range of services, autonomy, respect, provision of information, reliability, responsiveness, and cost.[19]

It would also be useful to survey for satisfaction beyond the patient level. The patient is defined as the consumer of home care, but there are many other customers who make decisions about the home care a patient will receive. These include both referral and payer sources. Information from these two areas will be helpful when looking at all aspects of an agency's performance.[20]

Existing Outcome-Measurement Systems

Outcome measurement in home care is in its early stages. There are several systems that have been developed over the years that have focused on the measurement of patient outcomes. These include the Omaha System for Community Health Nursing, Classifications of Home Health Nursing Diagnosis and Interventions, Wilson's Outcome Concepts System, and the Outcomes and Assessment Information Set (OASIS). Much of the current research has been focused on the OASIS system, since HCFA plans to use the results of these studies in the new requirements for Medicare-certified agencies.[21] Examination of the data elements used in these various systems can lead to a fuller understanding of what is currently being tracked and utilized in the home-care setting. The appendix lists a matrix of the data elements that are included in the various outcome systems in home care, and the data elements that are currently collected on the HCFA (Health Care Financing Agency) 485 and 486 patient-information forms.

The challenge of evaluating an outcome system for home health care includes identifying not only the predictor variables, but also the data elements that would make this outcome measure meaningful. Given that home-care nursing intervention has a significant impact on improving the functional status of the patient, an outcome measure that fails to evaluate functional status in the home-care patient will do little to demonstrate the effect of home-care nursing interventions.

Also key to making an outcome system meaningful is the ability of the data to be compared across settings. A number of agencies are already adapting or integrating OASIS with their current database systems. However, many agencies persist in using a variety of data-collection systems until the need for a universal outcome measure is acknowledged. A sample of outcome-measure systems that can form the basis for the development of a database in home care is reviewed in the following pages.

The Omaha System
The Omaha Visiting Nurses' Association (VNA) identified the need to develop a common language and an evaluation system for community-health nurses. The framework subsequently developed by the VNA is based on a blending of the nurse-patient relationship, nursing process, and the related theories of diagnostic reasoning and clinical judgment. The Omaha System is a taxonomy structured in three levels: problem-classification theme, intervention scheme, and problem-rating scale for outcomes.[22]

The problem-classification theme is divided into four different levels. Level One encompasses the domain of the patient, including environmental, psychological, physiological, and health-related problems. Level Two describes the patient problem with a listing of 40 nursing diagnoses. Level Three outlines health promotion, potential deficits, actual deficits, family, and individual characteristics. Lastly, Level Four is a listing of signs and symptoms, using a coding scheme for data-analysis purposes.[22] Expected outcomes and outcome criteria to be used by the home-health nurses in conjunction with the Problem Classification Scheme were also developed. The use of these outcomes enhance the effectiveness, accountability, and documentation of community-health nurses.

The Intervention Scheme is separated into hierarchical levels: categories, targets, and patient-specific information. Categories describe the primary functions of the nurse, encompassing health teaching, treatments and procedures, case management, and surveillance. The second level, targets, are the focus of the nursing interventions or activities. The third level, patient-specific information, is a documentation of pertinent information and planning of care for the individual patient. The Intervention Scheme is essentially a precise documentation of plans and interventions for patients.[22]

The last segment of the Omaha approach is the Problem Rating Scale for Outcomes, which is a systematic way to measure patient change. Patient problems are identified from a Problem Classification Scheme. Patient progress is measured and documented in relation to each problem on a Likert scale. Measurements of change should indicate whether interventions are effective and whether patient needs are being met.[22]

Home-Care Classification System
The Classifications of Home Health Nursing Diagnosis and Interventions (CHHN) were developed by Virginia Saba at Georgetown University as a language with which to assess and classify patients in order to determine the resources required to provide home-health services. The nursing diagnoses and interventions were grouped, classified, and coded using a framework of 20 Home Health Components. According to Saba, "A Home Health Nursing Component is defined as a cluster of elements that represents a health, functional, behavioral, or physiologic home health-care pattern. The twenty components provide the framework for assessing nursing service requirements, nursing diagnosis, expected outcomes/goals, nursing interventions and types of actions."[23]

In the classification of nursing interventions, four types of nursing actions were noted to occur: assessment, direct care, teaching, and management of services. Assessment actions included collection and analysis of data on the health status of patients. Direct care meant performing a therapeutic action. Teaching actions were providing knowledge and skill. The management of services involved coordinating and referring.[24]

These multiple levels of classification were then grouped in a format similar to, and therefore compatible with, the International Classification of Disease (ICD). This particular scheme of classification would enable coding to facilitate computer processing. Saba states that "these classifications offer an alternative approach for organizing the patient record, documenting the nursing process, and determining resource requirements." Perhaps most important is that the CHHN system provides data dictionaries for clinical nursing practice elements in computer-based patient record systems.[24]

Utilizing Saba's classification system would enhance the analysis of patient outcome measurement. It is not suggested that all of Saba's nursing interventions be included as specific data elements within a comprehensive database, although they could be included within a secondary database of nursing interventions. With this inclusion, nursing plans of care along with interventions could be an output option after keying in the other data elements.

Outcome Concepts System

Realizing the importance of functional status and the lack of accurate data describing or defining it, Wilson and Rinke developed a model of data collection, called the Outcome Concepts System (OCS), that integrates the functional status perspective into nursing documentation.[25] Using a functional status approach to define patient problems and outcomes, OCS creates a common language that is understood among health-care providers and consumers. It incorporates cost of care, patient satisfaction, and clinical goal in multiple formats.[26]

The outcome-measurement instrument presumes assessment of patient characteristics that are likely to be influenced by nursing: knowledge, skills, health, activities of daily living.[27] Using OCS, measurable changes in patient condition from admission to discharge can be analyzed. The functional status of each patient is weighted at admission and over time, until discharge.

Agencies using OCS are able to generate meaningful data on patient outcomes and use of services. The data collected in the OCS system will

- provide accurate statistical information to substantiate that quality care was provided;
- demonstrate how agency intervention affected the health and functional status of the patient;
- serve as a marketing tool for the agency; and
- provide data for the generation of internal and external agency reports.[26]

Perhaps the most attractive aspect of the OCS is the brevity of the assessment instrument. Wilson suggests that the employability of the data-collection tool is key to successful data collection.[26, 27] Completing outcomes-measurement tools can become an arduous chore for the home-care nurse. Efficient use of the nurses' time is critical in a growing industry, so usability of any instruments is a very important factor to consider.

OASIS

Medicare expenditures for home care account for approximately 9% of the total Medicare expenditures for health care, with the majority of health-care dollars being spent on hospital care.[13] Responsibility for the administration of the Medicare program falls under the auspices of the Health Care Finance Administration (HCFA). To ensure quality of care to Medicare recipients, as well as to maintain financial well-being, HCFA has been committed to the development of a patient-outcome measurement system that will help providers and payers predict patient needs, as well as interventions that will lead to desired outcomes.

Peter Shaughnessy and Kathryn Crisler of the Colorado Center for Health Policy and Services Research have made significant efforts to identify a conceptual framework and model around patient outcomes in home care. Their research was funded by the Health Care Financing Administration and the Robert Wood Johnson Foundation. Together, Shaughnessy and Crisler developed the Outcomes and Assessment Information Set (OASIS).[14]

The conceptual framework for OASIS is based on distinguishing an outcome from an outcome of care. "Outcomes," as has been stated, are changes in behavior. "Outcomes of care" implies an influence of interventions on the changes in behavior. Outcomes are placed into three categories: end-result outcome, intermediate-result outcome, and utilization outcome.[28]

The "end-result outcome" is defined as the change in health status between a baseline time point (admission) and a final time point (discharge). There is also qualification of antecedent care (provided by agency) and the natural progression of disease. If no care is provided, the disease will progress "naturally" (for better or worse). If health care is provided (agency-provided care for example), a resulting outcome will, hopefully, occur. The difference in the health status of the patient between the two time frames could be termed the "outcome of care."

HCFA has endorsed and encourages home-care agencies to use OASIS for Medicare recipients. Many agencies use some or all components of OASIS, and currently also collect additional data that meet the needs of other third-party payers. Data elements associated with hospice, pediatric, or maternity patients are not included in OASIS; therefore, adaptations must be made when assessing these patient populations. The developers of OASIS have recommended integration of the system with others where agencies serve more than just Medicare recipients. OASIS does not collect information specifically on nursing interventions, but instead is concerned with end-result outcomes, or the result of care provided by home-health nurses.[14] In addition, OASIS is designed in a Medicare framework, therefore it does not include data elements that relate to the care of children, maternal and prenatal care, or the care of hospice patients.

Currently, 50 Medicare-certified agencies are participating in a study testing the applicability of the OASIS instrument for home care. The purpose of this project is to establish a partnership between home-care agencies and the Medicare program in collecting and processing patient outcomes, improved agency performance, and a more efficient Medicare approach to quality improvement.[17]

Several variables are not included in the current OASIS format that may have a significant effect on the outcomes of care provided in the home. The impact of home-care interventions may be mediated by not assessing these areas and including them in the plan of care. The significant variables not included in the OASIS model are

- Religion/primary language spoken: Patient's culture and religion are factors which may reflect potential service use. The design of culturally sensitive services may require more or fewer visits by the home-care nurse or aide than indicated by a traditional care plan. For example, patients in certain cultures may be averse to having personal care provided by the home-health aide. This may require more home-care nursing visits to instruct the family on the personal care needed by the patient. The ability to effectively instruct patients on self care may be affected by their primary language.
- Literacy: A patient's ability to read the written word has significant implications for the amount and type of interventions provided by home care. In situations where literacy is compromised, the patient may require more frequent visits or visits of longer duration to teach self care.
- Visit level/resource utilization: A systematic record of resources employed per episode of home care provides data to monitor, evaluate, and predict use. Resources are defined as nursing and other disciplines intervening in the care of the patient or family, equipment, supplies, and time. Data elements would include discipline, number of visits, length of visit, equipment and supplies needed, and interventions provided. The intent is to relate a particular amount of effort or resources required to achieve desired outcomes in patient care. This information will facilitate billing, budgeting, and predicting needs, and enable strategic planning to meet those needs.

Summary

The science of outcome measurement as a method of assuring the quality of care provided has a firm grip on the home-care industry. Consumer demand, regulatory and payer requirements, and industry self-governance are all forces that will provide the fuel for continued development of methods to assess outcomes. As home care takes a preeminent place in the health-care delivery system, outcome measurement will provide the foundation for sound, clinical decision making, demonstrate the value of home care to the health and well-being of patients, and facilitate the development of relationships across the health-care continuum.

Home-health agencies are challenged to measure, evaluate, and validate their services and their impact on the individual's and the nation's health. Without reliable data, it is impossible to achieve such a mission. Research in the area of home-health services is needed to describe and predict home health-care use. Data is needed for analysis of resource allocation, assurance of quality, and the determination of cost in planning for public policy making.

References

1. C. Adams and M. Wilson, "Enhanced Quality Through Outcome Focused Standardized Care Plan," *Journal of Nursing Administration* (1995): 25(9):27—34.
2. J. Mefford, "Order in a New Era: Outcome Documentation," *Caring* (1996): 15(6):18—20.
3. K.N. Lohr, K. Yordy, P.F. Garrison, and A.C. Gelijns, "Health Care Systems: Lessons From International Comparisons," *Health Affairs* (1992): 11(4):239—41.
4. K. Carney, "The Physician's Perspective on Home Care," *Caring* (1996): 15(4):14—19.
5. A. Kolatch, "Marketing Home Health Care," *Journal of Nursing Administration* (1991): 21(11):52.
6. C. Schaffer and F. Srp, "Outcome Driven Home Care," *Caring* (1996): 15(6):8—12.
7. American Managed Care and Review Association Foundation, *Managed Care Overview* (Washington, DC: Author, 1994—95), 78.
8. E. Eckholm, "While Congress Remains Silent, Health Care Transforms Itself," New York *Times*, Sunday, December 18, 1994.
9. R. Fazzi and R. Agoglia, "What Home Care Executives Should Know About Managed Care Organizations: Preliminary Results From a National Study," *Caring* (1995): 10(2):78—85.
10. National Association for Home Care, "A United Home Care Industry Proposes Prospective Payment for Medicare Home Health Services as a Substitute for Copays and Bundling," *NAHC Report* 654a, 1996.
11. K. G. Manton, M. A. Woodbury, J. C. Vertrees, and E. Stallard, "Use of Medicare Services Before and after Introduction of the Prospective Payment System," *Health Services Research* (1993): 28(3):269—92.
12. P.A. Dee-Kelly, S. Heller, and M. Sibley, "Managed Care: An Opportunity for Home Care Agencies," *Nursing Clinics of North America* (1994): 29(3):471-81.
13. National Association for Home Care, *Basic Statistics About Home Care 1996* (Washington, DC: National Association for Home Care).
14. P. Shaughnessy, K. Crisler, R. Schlenker, A. Arnold, A. Kramer, M. Powell, and D. Hittle, "Measuring and Assuring the Quality of Home Health Care," *Health Care Financing Review* (1994): 16(1):35—65.
15. C. Woodham-Smith, *Florence Nightingale 1820—1910* (London: Constable and Co., 1950).
16. P.A. Prescott, K.L. Soeken, and M. Griggs, "Identification and Referral of Hospitalized Patients in Need of Home Care," *Research in Nursing and Health Care* (1995): 18:85—95.
17. M. Seago and C. Conn, "Outcome Based Quality Improvement Documentation," *Caring* (1996): 15(6):67.
18. J. Williams, "Measuring Outcomes in Home Care: Current Research and Practice," *Health Care Services Quarterly* (1995): 15(3):3—30.
19. M.E. Henry and H. Capitman, *A Providers Guide to Assessing Consumer Satisfaction* (Waltham, MA: Brandeis University, 1995).
20. M.B. Peterson, "Measuring Patient Satisfaction: Collecting Useful Data," *Journal of Nursing Quality Assurance* (1988): 2(3):25—35.

21. National Association for Home Care, "Outcomes: Answering Questions About Home Care," *Caring* (1996): 15(6):7.
22. K.S. Martin and N.J. Scheet, *The Omaha System: Applications for Community Health Nursing* (Philadelphia: W.B. Saunders, 1992).
23. V.K. Saba, "The Classification of Home Care Nursing Diagnoses and Interventions," *Caring* (1992): 11(3):8—9, 50—57.
24. V.K. Saba, "The Classification of Home Health Nursing Diagnoses and Interventions." *HHCC Project Report for Health Care Finance Administration* (Washington, DC: Georgetown University School of Nursing, 1990), 8.
25. A. Wilson and L. Rinke, "DRGs and the Measurement of Quality in Home Care," *Nursing Clinics of North America* (1988): 23(3):569—78.
26. A. Wilson, "The Quest for Accountability: Patient Costs and Outcomes," *Caring* (1996): 15(6):24—29.
27. A.A. Wilson, "The Cost and Quality of Patient Outcomes," *Nursing Administration Quarterly* (1993): 17(4):11—16.
28. P. Shaughnessy and K. Crisler, *Outcome-Based Quality Improvement: A Manual for Home Care Agencies on How to Use Outcomes* (Denver: Colorado Center for Health Policy and Services Research, National Association for Home Care, 1995).

Measurement of Outcomes in Home Care: An Overview

APPENDIX A

Table 1
Matrix of Common Information Collected

ELEMENT	OASIS	CHHN	OMAHA	OCS	HCFA (485 & 486 forms)
Demographics	x	x	x	x	x
Allergies	x	x			
Diagnosis & Prognosis					
Inpatient Discharge within 14 days	x	x			
Inpatient Discharge Date	x	x	x		
Inpatient Diagnosis	x	x			
Medical Regimen Change within past 14	x				
Changed Medical Regimen DX (ICD)	x	x			
Conditions Prior to Medical Regimen Ch	x				
Primary Diagnosis (ICD)	x	x	x		
Severity Index	x				
Therapies	x				
Overall Prognosis	x		x	x	
Rehabilitative Prognosis	x	x	x		
Life Expectancy	x	x			
High Risk Factors	x	x	*		
Surgical Procedures	x	*	x		
Nursing Diagnosis	x	x			
Antepartum/Postpartum	x				
Physiological Status					
Vision	x	x	x	x	
Hearing	x	x	x	x	
Speech/Oral Expression	x	x	x	x	
Pain	x	x	x	x	
Intractable Pain	x	x	x		
Integumentary (Main Heading in Oasis)	x	x	x	x	
Open Wound	x	x	*		
Pressure Ulcers	x	x	*		
Most Problematic Ulcer	x	x	*		
Wounds Present	x	x	*	x	
Wound/Lesion Status	x	x	*		
Dyspnea	x	x	x	x	x
Treatments	x	x	*	x	

Table 1 (continued)
Matrix of Common Information Collected

ELEMENT	OASIS	CHHN	OMAHA	OCS	HCFA (485 & 486 forms)
Genitourinary Status (major category of OASIS)	x	x	x	x	
UTI	x	x	*		
Urinary Incontinence or Catheter Presen	x	x	x	x	x
Bowel Incontinence	x	x	x	x	
Ostomy	x	x	*		
Musculoskeletal	x	x	x		
Cardiovascular Status	x	x	x		
Nutrition Status	x	x	x	x	
Fluid Volume	x	x			
Physical Regulation	x	x			
Role Relationship	x	x			
Tissue Perfusion	x	x			
Psychological Status					
Neurologic Status (Main Category)	x	x	*	x	
Cognitive Functioning	x	x	x	x	
When Confused	x	x	*		
Depressive Feelings	x	x	*	x	
Behaviors Observed	x	x	*		
Behaviors Demonstrated	x	x	*		
Behavior Problem Frequency	x	x	*		
Psychiatric Nursing Services	x	x			
Functional Status					
Grooming	x	x	x	x	
Dress Upper Body	x	x	*	x	
Dress Lower Body	x	x	*	x	
Bathing	x	x	*	x	
Toileting	x	x	*	x	
Transferring	x	x	x	x	x
Ambulation/Locomotion	x	x	x	x	x
Feeding/eating	x	x	*	x	
Planning and Preparing Light Meals	x	x	x		
Transportation	x	x			
Laundry	x	x			
Housekeeping	x	x			
Shopping	x	x			
Ability to use Telephone	x	x			
Management of Oral Medications	x	x	x	x	x

Measurement of Outcomes in Home Care: An Overview **17**

Table 1 (continued)
Matrix of Common Information Collected

ELEMENT	OASIS	CHHN	OMAHA	OCS	HCFA (485 & 486 forms)
Management of Inhalant/ Mist Medication					
Management of Injectable Medications	x	x	*	x	
Safety	x	x	x	x	
Functional Limitations/ Reason Homebound/ Prior status	*		x		
Unusual Home/Social Environment		x			
Discharge Info					
D/C, Transfer, Death Data	x	x			
D/C Disposition	x	x			
Reason for D/C	*	x			
Services Patient Receiving in Community	x	x			
Reason for Hospitalization	x				
Reason for NHP Using Home Placement	x				
Providers Name	x		x		
Date Physician Last Saw Patient		x			
Date Last Contacted Physician	*		x		
Discharge Service Provided	x	x			
Service Data					
Reason for Leaving home		x			
Time When Patient Not Home		x			
Date of Visit	*				
Type of Visit	*				
Escorted/Non-escorted/ DBL Escorted					
Interpreted/Noninterpreted					
Joint Visit with Others					
Durable Medical Equipment and Supplies	x	x			
Identify PT Nursing Need (Type, Intervention, Action)	x	*			
Assess Direct Care, Educate, MGT of Services	x				
Nursing Intervention	x	*			
ICD-9 Codes of Procedures Performed	x				

Table 1 (continued)
Matrix of Common Information Collected

ELEMENT	OASIS	CHHN	OMAHA	OCS	HCFA (485 & 486 forms)
HCPCS Codes of Procedures Performed					
Resolution of Outcomes	x	x			
Length of Visits	x				
Minutes of Service Traveled					
Unit of Service Visit					
Unit of Service per Discipline					
Number of Days per Hospice Care					

X *Exact information collected*
* *Similar, but not exact information collected*

About the Authors

Dr. Paula Milone-Nuzzo has over 15 years' experience as a home-care provider, manager, educator, and consultant. She is currently on the faculty of Yale University School of Nursing, where she is an associate professor and chair of the Specialty Care and Management Division. She is responsible for teaching masters and doctoral students in her course, Advanced Concepts in Home Care. She has provided consultation to numerous home-care agencies on issues of quality improvement, strategic planning, and joint venturing.

Milone-Nuzzo is nationally and internationally known for her writing and speaking on orientation to home-care nursing. Her many publications deal with all aspects of home health-care delivery from advanced clinical practice to the management of home-care delivery systems. Milone-Nuzzo is involved in research which examines the effect of home-care interventions on the cost and quality of care provided to repeat users of emergency-room service. She was an investigator in a project that resulted in the development of a computerized documentation system for home-health aides.

Dr. Milone-Nuzzo sits on numerous boards, having a leadership position in both local and state home-care activities.

Susan Brink, Julu Huang, Karen Levine, and Moira O'Neill are all students in the Nursing Management and Policy Program at Yale University School of Nursing, designed to prepare nursing leaders in the area of health policy and management. Students are required to participate in a project identified by and of value to a health-care agency. The foundation for this monograph was the work done by these students on the development of a database system for the Connecticut Association for Home Care.

Chapter 2

OUTCOME DATA ANALYSIS: PUTTING RESULTS INTO PRACTICE

by Jan Herzog, MSN, RN, Clinical Program Development Analyst and Mary Schoen, MSN, MPH, RN, Director of Education Services
The Visiting Nurse Association of Greater Philadelphia

Abstract

Health-care reform and the move to provide more cost-efficient services are having a significant impact on home-health nursing practice. Using the results of outcome-based studies and utilization of nursing resources, the Visiting Nurse Association of Greater Philadelphia restructured their hiring, orientation, and training programs for the nursing staff. Clinical competencies are defined to ensure that the nurses are clinically skilled and highly knowledgeable to deliver effective patient care in today's rapidly changing home healthcare environment. They conclude with examples of the tools used in this process.

Outcome Data Analysis: Putting Results Into Practice

Sitting at the edge of a new millennium probably provides no better time than to reflect on the tremendous expansion occurring in the home health-care field. In 1963, there were some 1,100 home-care agencies. Their numbers grew to 11, 097 by 1989, and to more than 18, 500 home-care agencies currently.[1] Today, home-care providers deliver home-care services to some seven million individuals who require such services because of acute illness, long-term health conditions, permanent disability, or terminal illness.

With the rapid growth of the home-care industry, home-care nursing practice is undergoing radical changes. Home-care nurses now use technology that once only existed in intensive care units. Nurses are instructing patients and their caregivers how to manage ventilators, ambulatory dialysis, and continuous infusion of medications. Innovative home-based programs, such as cardiac recovery programs for coronary artery bypass graft (CABG) surgery and crisis intervention for psychiatric patients have added new sophistication to home care. As a result, acutely ill home-health patients require both acute-care and home health-care nursing skills.[2]

Another significant impact on home-care nursing practice is health-care reform and the move to more cost-efficient services. Although home-care services are highly valued and cost effective, the industry must be able to quantify the care delivered in the home. The home-care agency must show progressive documentation not only of the care provided, but also must indicate that patient outcomes were achieved within a certain period of time. Without the essential documentation, home-care agencies will not be able to compete in the current health-care market. As consumers of health care, managed-care companies comparison shop when determining who will receive contracts to provide home-care services for their members. Managed-care companies are looking for the best buys for their money.

To meet the demands of a medically complex home-care population and a changing health-care environment, it is obvious that a home-care agency's training program must be refined to ensure that the nurses are clinically skilled and highly effective in delivering positive patient outcomes. The following pages describe how the Visiting Nurse Association of Greater Philadelphia (VNAGP) used the results of outcome-data analysis and resource-utilization measures to structure the agency's hiring, orientation, and training programs for the nursing staff.

Background
The VNAGP, founded in 1886, is one of the oldest and largest regional providers of home-health services in the Delaware Valley. Last year, the VNAGP provided a half-million visits to patients of all ages living in Philadelphia and the surrounding counties. The VNAGP is a multispecialty agency and offers a wide range of programs such as infusion therapy, hospice, mental health services, a high risk infant and pre-natal program, continence care, and a wound/ostomy program. In response to market demand, the VNAGP recently developed an oncology specialty program and a cardio-pulmonary care program. All of the specialty programs are led by advanced-practice nurses and staffed with clinicians proficient in the particular specialization. In developing the competencies for the specialty programs, the VNAGP needed to define those competencies necessary for the generalist nurse.

Role of the Home Health-Care Nurse
Although there is a great deal of similarity between the nursing practice of home health-care nurses and their colleagues who work in a hospital, there are many roles that a home health-care nurse must assume that are different. A review of the literature reveals a wealth of information regarding the skills and knowledge needed in home health care.[3-7] Table 1 defines the major job elements found to be critical to productive nurse practice in home health care.

Table 1
Home-Care Nursing Skills and Knowledge

Assessment	Proficiency in medical surgical nursing procedures
	Perform general psychophysiologic assessments that apply across the life span
	Self-directed, flexible, and able to practice independently
	Ability to assess the home environment
Case Management	Excellent interpersonal skills—both written and oral
	A working knowledge of community resources
	Interdisciplinary communication skills
	Knowledge of state, federal, and accrediting-body requirements
Teaching	Teaching ability
	Knowledge of principles of adult learning

These core competencies can be grouped into three major categories: assessment, case management, and teaching. The three core components are included in the VNAGP's basic orientation program and further enhanced in the agency's specialty training programs.

The practice of home-health nursing is focused predominantly on the care of individuals, in collaboration with the family and designated caregivers. Practice activities center on secondary prevention (treatment, care, rehabilitation), assistance to families, and coordination of community resources.

All nursing care is based on a complete physical, psychosocial, and environmental assessment. Data collection is an essential prerequisite to the assessment of the individual and the family. The process allows the nurse to reach sound conclusions and plan interventions based in both scientific and social theories.[8]

The home-care nurse also functions as the coordinator of services required to achieve the desired outcomes. Case-management activities demand sound decision-making and priority-setting skills. Without specific nursing intervention, gaps and fragmentation occur in the delivery of health-care services, causing the patient's condition to be compromised. The home-care nurse is responsible for working with all members of the health-care team to ensure that everyone involved is working towards the same patient-care outcomes.

The third critical component of home-care practice involves patient and caregiver education. Teaching activities focus on instructions for self-care activities that are necessary to achieve and maintain wellness and prevent complications. Patient outcomes are usually defined using the results of the teaching performed. To achieve positive patient outcomes, patients and their caregivers require a thorough understanding of the health problems and how to successfully manage them.

Outcome Measurement in Home Health Care

The current focus on patient outcomes is a result of health-care economics, specifically the need for cost-effective care in the managed health-care environment.[9] The emerging science of outcome measurement has the potential to impact positively on patient care. Shaughnessey and Crisler defined a patient outcome as a change in patient health status between two or more time points.[10] The change can be positive, neutral, or negative, and can occur either as a result of the care provided or in the natural progression of disease and disability. Patient outcome data must adequately and consistently measure quality. Information on patient outcomes is essential for directing an agency's evaluation-of-care process, which can lead to improvement in services.

Outcome Concept System

The VNAGP uses the Outcome Concept System (OCS), which was developed by Alexis Wilson to measure patient outcomes.[11] The OCS national network represents the largest group of home health-care providers using one uniform data-collection mechanism. OCS is one of the leading sources of aggregate data on outcomes in the United States. The VNAGP uses OCS to measure changes in health and functional status for patients with the medical diagnoses of congestive health failure (CHF), cerebrovascular accident (CVA), diabetes, asthma, and cancer. These five diagnostic groups represent approximately 40% of patients admitted for service.

Four functional status categories are used to compare patient outcomes at the time of admission and at the time of discharge from home-care service. Table 2 describes the functional categories.

Table 2
OCS Functional Categories

Health status	Patient's physiological condition
Skill function	Ability of the patient or caregiver to perform tasks and activities necessary to restore or maintain health
Knowledge function	Evaluates what the patient or caregiver needs to know to safely manage care within the limits of their ability
Psychosocial function	Ability to cope with the demands imposed by the health-care problems

The ratings for the OCS tools are divided into four categories: 25%—the lowest level, 50%, 75% and 100%—the highest level (*see* Appendix 1). The system quantifies changes in health and functional status as a result of care provided. It measures what happened as a result of nursing interventions. Managed-care companies are beginning to request the VNAGP's outcome data. With the outcome system that the VNAGP is currently using, the agency is moving towards providing this type of data.

Outcome Data Analysis
On a quarterly basis, patient data is manually entered into the OCS database. Data, obtained from patient discharge records for that quarter, include social security number, name, address, gender, date of birth, admission and discharge dates and reason, payer referral source, primary physician, ADL status, and number of visits per discipline.

The VNAGP uses the reports and graphs describing the following.

- Distribution of Services: percent of service delivered by each discipline involved in the patient's care
- Functional Status: functional status at the time of admission and discharge for health, knowledge, skill, and psychosocial function
- Functional Change: the change (maintaining, improving, declining) from admission to discharge in the four functional categories
- Special Items: discharge reason, length of stay, and cost analysis

Outcome Data Results
Through analysis of the patient outcome data and associated clinical interventions, VNAGP staff identified the following areas for improvement in nursing practice.

- Patient assessments that are clinically consistent with patient's medical condition
- Identification of key nursing interventions for specific medical problems
- Improve patient teaching methods and materials on how to perform skills and self-care tasks in the home setting
- Need for better management of acutely ill patients
- A documentation system that would provide prompts and cues for patient assessments and interventions

Identification of areas for improvement prompted the VNAGP to act in two ways. The first step was to upgrade the VNAGP's training program to ensure that staff were clinically competent to meet the demands of patients who were being discharged from acute-care facilities into the home, "sicker and quicker." The second action was to develop disease-specific clinical pathways.

Training Programs

Recruitment and Hiring

A home-health agency's first challenge is to recruit and hire nurses with the appropriate credentials and skills. At the VNAGP, the majority of nurses applying for employment have no home health-care experience. Many nurses laid off from acute-care hospitals apply to the VNAGP for employment. Fortunately, many nurses are coming with excellent assessment skills.

The VNAGP uses several methods in the hiring process to ascertain previous experience in specialty areas. First, all new applicants complete a self-assessment skills checklist to evaluate their knowledge in critical job elements. The checklist includes critical skills needed for a more acutely ill home health-care population. It is used to obtain a baseline assessment of competence from the employee's perspective. Employees rank their clinical skills as very experienced, somewhat experienced, or not experienced. The self-assessment assists the VNAGP in determining if the nurse possesses the knowledge base and clinical skills necessary to safely care for the patient population to which they will be assigned. In hiring for the disease-specific programs, the VNAGP further evaluates staff by looking for certification from national organizations and evidence of continuing education in the particular specialty.

General Orientation

The VNAGP's orientation program uses Knowles' theory, which states that adult learners bring previous knowledge which should be built on rather than retaught.[12] The process uses competency-based outcome modules that describe specific objectives for knowledge and skill acquisition (see Appendix 2). The orientation is a blending of formalized instruction, self-directed learning, and one-on-one mentoring in the clinical setting. Particular attention is paid to the new employee's assessment and patient teaching skills.

Nurses complete the general orientation program to ensure competence in providing nursing services in the home setting. Competence is defined as the demonstration of knowledge and skills in meeting professional role expectations.[13] The orientation program is closely modeled on the standards outlined in the "Management of Human Resources" section of the *Joint Commission Standards for Home Health Care*.[14] Close supervision and targeted program content prepare new home-health nurses for competent practice in highly independent roles, reduce legal and professional risk, and make reasonable use of supervisory time and effort needed to ensure safe practice. Joint home visits are made with all new staff to ensure competence in the performance of home-care nursing interventions.

Specialty Training Programs

Once the general competence in providing home health-care service is confirmed, the specialty nurse can advance to the next educational level—the opportunity to become a member of the specialty program which incorporates the knowledge and skills of the nurse's area of clinical expertise. This process usually takes place about six months to one year following initial employment.

The VNAGP employs advanced practice nurses to assist in providing care to increasingly complex and highly technical patient populations. The Advanced Practice Nurse (APN) is a master's-prepared nurse who, through study and supervised practice, has become an expert in a selected area of nursing practice.[15] The APN functions as a resource person in the form of an expert consultant and educator.

The APN presents specialty training classes for specialty teams. The training program includes education on the etiology and demographics of the specific disease process, normal and abnormal physiology, risk factors, diagnostic tests, medical and nursing interventions, medication management, identification and management of complications, patient-education materials, and community resources. At the end of the didactic classes, participants take a comprehensive examination. The training includes joint home visits to allow the APN to evaluate the nurses on the clinical competencies related to the area of specialty practice. Upon successful completion of the specialty training course, the nurse is awarded a "certificate of competency" from the agency.

Continuing Education

The VNAGP implemented a skills lab to provide all nursing staff with the additional skills necessary to care for their "sicker" patients. The purpose of the skills lab is to develop and enhance home-health nurses' competencies relative to the changing technology in the home-care environment. Skills were selected based on their clinical significance to the patient population (Doppler and Pulse Oximeter), and low-frequency skills (male and female catheterization, tracheostomy care). Glucose monitoring was added, as the JCAHO requires that an annual competency evaluation be performed.

Skill stations are set up in a large conference room and manned by nurses from each of the specialty programs. At each station, a mannequin or piece of equipment is provided for nurses to demonstrate their competency. Several of the stations include self-learning packets which staff complete during the laboratory time. Nurses work at their own pace in a relaxed learning atmosphere. A skills checklist is completed for each skill demonstrated correctly. This checklist is filed in the employee's personnel record as documentation of skill competency. The skills laboratory exposes staff members to equipment and procedures many never used or performed. It expands staff nurses' clinical knowledge base and increases confidence in providing services to patients.

References

1. V.J. Halamandaris, *Basic Statistics about Home Care* (Washington, DC: National Association for Home Care, 1996).
2. V. Kenyon, E. Smith, L.V. Hefty, et. al., "Clinical Competencies for Community Health Nursing," *Public Health Nursing* (1990): 7(1):33—39.
3. L.W. Smith, "Designing Training Programs for Specialty Services," *Caring* (1996): 25(5):42-45.
4. L.V. Hefty, V. Kenyon, T. Martaus, et. al., "A Model Skills List for Orienting Nurses to Community Health Agencies," *Public Health Nursing* (1992): 9(4):228—33.
5. T.A. Murray, "Switching from Hospital-Based Practice to Home Care," *Home Care Provider* (1996): 1(2):79—82.
6. C.J. Humphrey and P. Milone-Nuzzo, "Home Care Nursing Orientation Model: Justification and Structure," *Home Health Care Nurse* (1992): 10:18—25.
7. T.M. Astarita, "Competency-Based Orientation in Home Health Care: One Agency's Approach," *Home Health Care Management & Practice* (1996): 8(4):38—49.
8. American Nurses Association, *Standards of Home Health Nursing Practice* (Kansas City, MO: The American Nurses Association, 1986).
9. B. Jennings, "Patient Outcomes Research: Seizing the Opportunity," *Advances in Nursing Science* (1991): 14(2):59—72.
10. P. Shaughnessy and K. Crisler, *Outcome-Based Quality Improvement* (Washington, DC: National Association for Home Care, 1995).
11. A. Wilson and M. Hartnett, *Outcome Concept Systems: A Guide to Measurement of Patient Outcome* (Gig Harbor, WA: Wilson & Associates, 1996).
12. M.S. Knowles, *The Modern Practice of Adult Education: Andragogy versus Pedagogy* (New York Association Press, 1980).
13. American Nurses Association, *Standards for Nursing Professional Development, Continuing Education and Staff Development* (Washington, DC: American Nurses Publishing, 1994).
14. Joint Commission on Accreditation of Health Care Organizations, *Accreditation Standards for Home Health Care Education and Training* (Oakbrook Terrace, IL: 1994).
15. L. Neal, "The Clinical Nurse Specialist: Practice in the Home Health Care Setting," *Home Health Care Management & Practice* (1996): 8(3):64—68.
16. V. Mauren and L. Van Dyck, "Using Outcome Based Critical Pathways to Improve Documentation," *Home Health Care Management & Practice* (1996): 8(2):48—58.

APPENDIX A

Visiting Nurse Association of Greater Philadelphia
Patient Outcomes

Patient Name: _____ Stat #: _____

Complete at the time of <u>admission, recert, and discharge.</u>

	25%	50%	75%	100%
KNOWLEDGE Ability to remember and interpret instructions	Verbalizes no apparent knowledge	Verbalizes minimal knowledge	Verbalizes substantial knowledge	Verbalizes competent knowledge
	Adm: _____	Recert: _____	D/C: _____	
SKILL Ability to perform skills/procedures	Demonstrates no skill	Demonstrates minimal skill	Demonstrates substantial skill	Demonstrates competent skill
	Adm: _____	Recert: _____	D/C: _____	
HEALTH STATUS Patient's condition	Declining	Stable	Improving	Problem resolved
	Adm: _____	Recert: _____	D/C: _____	
COPING BEHAVIOR Ability to adapt to lifestyle changes	No apparent self-esteem/ motivation	Low self-esteem/ motivation	Adequate self-esteem/ motivation	High self-esteem/ motivation
	Adm: _____	Recert: _____	D/C: _____	

VN Signature: _____ Date: _____

Outcome Concept System rating scale reprinted with permission of The Visiting Nurse Association of Greater Philadelphia.

APPENDIX B

**VNA of Greater Philadelphia
Competency-Based Orientation
Adult Health**

Upon completion of orientation the RN will be able to:

Competency Statement	Resources	Evaluation Mechanism	Date Met
Verbalize VNA organizational structure/mission/vision	organizational chart	verbal feedback	_____
Identify components of the Home Care Record	Education Coordinator	return demonstration	_____
Identify strategies to minimize safety risks in the community	Education Coordinator; *Street Smarts* video	verbal feedback	_____
Identify signs and symptoms of abuse in children and the elderly	Education Coordinator; *Elder Abuse* video	competency test	_____
Summarize the following VNA Policies: a) Patient Rights & Responsibilities b) Confidentiality c) Admission & D/C Criteria d) Dress Code e) Incident Reporting f) Patient Education g) Home Safety	Policy Manual	competency test	_____
Identify the information to be reported to the pre-cert nurses	Education Coordinator	verbal feedback	_____
Understand OSHA regulations and infection-control policies	Infection-Control Coordinator; *Infection Control* video	verbal feedback	_____
Document to meet JCAHO standards and federal regulations	Education Coordinator	return demonstration	_____
Successfully conduct a home visit	Patient-Care Manager	field visit tool	_____
Understand the role of the Patient-Care Manager: Supervisory Visits Patient Coverage Documentation Review	Education Coordinator	verbal feedback	_____

Annual Performance Review Case Conferences			

Understand the role of:
  Nutritionist
  Psychiatric Nurse
  ET Nurse
  Social Work
  Home-health Aide
  Rehab Staff
	Policy Manual:
	Guidelines for
	Referral
		verbal feedback	_____

Identify mandatory inservice education requirements	inservice education policy; Education Coordinator	verbal feedback	_____
Employee Signature:		Date:	
Education Coordinator Signature:		Date:	

Competency-based orientation checklist reprinted with permission of The Visiting Nurse Association of Greater Philadelphia.

About the Authors

Jan Herzog, MSN, RN, is the Clinical Program Development Analyst at The Visiting Nurse Association of Greater Philadelphia. She has over ten years of extensive administrative and clinical experience in home health care. Current responsibilities at the VNAGP include the development and implementation of disease management programs, including analysis of patient outcomes using the Outcome Concept System. She has been actively involved in the staff education programs related to disease management, clinical pathways, and patient outcomes. Herzog received her MSN from the University of Pennsylvania, BSN from Wichita State University, and ADN from the University of South Dakota.

Mary Schoen, MSN, MPH, RN, is the Director of Education Services at The Visiting Nurse Association of Greater Philadelphia. She started her career in home health care with the Visiting Nurse Service of New York in 1981. She held a variety of positions with the agency, including staff nurse, orientation nurse, and patient-service manager. In 1989, Mary joined New York City's Health and Hospitals Corporation as a senior program planner for the municipal hospitals' home health-care agencies. In her current position as Director of Education Services for the VNA of Greater Philadelphia, Schoen is administratively responsible for a staff development program that supports the orientation, inservice, and continuing-education needs of clinical and non-clinical staff. Schoen received her joint MS in nursing and public health from Columbia University. She received her BSN from New York University in 1980.

Chapter 3

CRITICAL PATHWAYS DEFINE BEST PRACTICE

by Joanne M. Rokosky, MN, RNCS, *Clinical and Staff Development Specialist*
Cynthia Drucker, BA, CPHQ, *Quality Improvement Manager*
and Joanne Ozaki-Moore, MEd, BSN, *Patient Services Manager*
Visiting Nurse Services of the Northwest

Abstract

Visiting Nurse Services of the Northwest (VNS-NW) is committed to the challenge of determining how to most effectively allocate resources to achieve positive patient outcomes. As one approach to this challenge, the agency developed a new documentation system based on its definition of "best practice" as patient care that is of high quality, focused toward outcomes, and cost effective. Two complementary components of this documentation system were developed in tandem: a) diagnosis-specific critical pathways, referred to as VNS-NW Pathways to Health©, and b) a generic critical pathway referred to as Outcome Based Documentation System (OBDS). Both types of critical pathways systematically shifted the documentation focus toward clear identification of patient problems, determination of realistic patient outcomes, and choice of clinician interventions most likely to achieve these outcomes. Clinician feedback and analysis of initial outcome data led to development of additional strategies needed to achieve "best practice." The long-term goal is to better target clinician and visit resources toward realistic outcomes.

Introduction

In this time of intense and aggressive competition for market share, home-health agencies (HHA) must analyze the efficiency of resource allocation and determine which patient outcomes can reasonably be achieved through clinician interventions. Campbell challenges the home-care industry to "look forward and out, instead of focusing down and inward."[1] HHAs must design economical delivery systems and be prepared for ongoing re-examination and re-design to meet market demands.

Visiting Nurse Services of the Northwest (VNS-NW) is committed to the challenge of defining and re-defining how to effectively allocate resources to achieve positive patient outcomes. This article describes how VNS-NW defined "best practice" as patient care that is of high quality, focused toward positive outcomes, and cost effective. This best practice definition is the basis for guiding the agency toward improvements in clinical practice and documentation.

Impetus for Change
VNS-NW is a large, freestanding home-health agency located in the Pacific Northwest. Home-health and hospice visits are made from branch offices located in three contiguous counties. In addition to providing intermittent home health care, the agency offers hourly professional and non-professional services and a clinic program with affiliations in numerous community sites.

By the fall of 1993, managed care began to impact the Northwest. Its advent necessitated that clinicians focus interventions toward measurable patient outcomes achievable in a limited number of visits.[2] The predicted shift in Medicare reimbursement further supported the need to better target clinician and visit resources toward realistic outcomes. Unfortunately, the agency's documentation did not lend itself to new ways of thinking, planning care, and structuring visits. For example, the format for home-visit documentation was largely narrative, and contained few printed cues linking it to the initial plan of care. Chart audits confirmed that numerous goals identified at admission were not addressed during the episode of care.

The documentation system clearly needed revision. Three assumptions guided the documentation revision process at VNS-NW. First, changes must be agency-wide and eliminate segments of documentation that differed among branch offices. Second, clinicians must be integral partners in development. Third, cohesiveness and collaboration between clinicians and managers within and between geographic sites must result.

Changing the plan of care and integrating critical pathways into home health were identified as the priorities for documentation revision. The plan of care needed to link patient problems and expected patient/patient-caregiver outcomes with clinician interventions. Although in its most basic form a critical pathway only plots interventions or tasks against a time frame, more comprehensive pathways include a list of patient problems, expected patient outcomes, and a variance record.[3] Thus, development of critical pathways meshed well with the plan of care changes. In addition, critical pathways offered a system to track variance and categorize the reasons for failure to achieve outcomes. These variance data would be useful internally to examine patient mix and negotiate contracts. Externally, the variance data would justify to payers and referral sources the need for additional visits to complicated patients.[4]

Development of Critical Pathways

VNS-NW began developing home-health critical pathways by analyzing the patient population. Patient demographic characteristics, length of home-health admission, the number of visits made per discipline, and supply costs were determined for 61 ICD-9 diagnoses. Data from 10,000 patients collected over three consecutive 12-month periods were analyzed.

VNS-NW focused pathway development on high-volume primary diagnoses. Work began with a relatively simple medical diagnosis, then progressed to the complicated problems more characteristic of home health. The initial target diagnosis was acute wound. The second target was the considerably more complex diagnosis of congestive heart failure (CHF).

Initial Pathway Development. Development of the first two pathways began with retrospective chart reviews to capture detailed baseline data about patient characteristics and clinician practice patterns. Open abdominal wounds, ICD-9 879, were selected to represent the acute-wound diagnosis. The complexity of this patient population, believed to represent the most straightforward patient group within the agency, was surprising. Patients had co-existing secondary medical diagnoses contributing to immunosuppression and delayed healing, functional limitations, and socioeconomic complications. The wounds themselves were invariably complicated; many required irrigation and extensive packing. Similarly, charts were reviewed for patients with congestive heart failure, ICD-9 428. This review again revealed the complex nature of the patients. For example, each patient had three to eight co-morbid diagnoses and an average of nine different medications.

The retrospective reviews were assigned to the nursing clinicians comprising the respective acute-wound and CHF pathway work groups. One intent of this assignment was to stimulate clinicians to discuss practice variations among the four geographic sites. The hope was that an open discussion would promote development of cohesive groups focused on identifying "best practice" for the whole agency.

Again, the result was a surprise. Clinicians did not discern characteristic patterns of practice among offices. Instead, practice patterns were unique to individual clinicians and reflected variable practice levels and adherence to agency standards. For example, the acute-wound-care review revealed that some clinicians documented according to the agency-wide wound-care protocol, while others did not. The clinicians uniformly observed that documentation was inadequate.

Clearly, "best practice" needed to be built from the ground up, using clinician experience and literature findings. To start this process, we compared patient data and visit patterns within VNS-NW to recommendations contained in two home-health critical-pathway products, CareMaps® (now called Home

Care Steps™) and Milliman and Robertson Home Care and Case Management Guidelines. Neither product matched the VNS-NW patient population or agency direction. Consequently, the agency proceeded with development of its own system.

Developing the first two pathways, Acute Wound and CHF, was circuitous and slow. Expected patient outcomes, clinical interventions, standards of practice, and documentation format were subjects of spirited debate. The intense, forceful interchanges clarified practice expectations and led to development of a standardized documentation template that objectified the components of "best practice."

Ongoing Pathway Development. For subsequent pathways, in-depth retrospective chart review was discontinued on the assumption that enough was known to predict the findings: complicated patients with many co-morbidities and no predictable pattern of clinician practice. The basic process for pathway development was maintained, but accelerated. Clinician input was limited to outlining the standards of "best practice" related to each pathway diagnosis. Clinical managers used the results of clinician brainstorming to complete the development of each subsequent pathway. To date, the following additional pathways have been completed for nursing: Pressure Ulcer, Venous Stasis Ulcer, Coronary Artery Bypass Graft, and Chronic Obstructive Pulmonary Disease (COPD). Diabetes Mellitus is near completion. Occupational therapy and social-work clinicians drafted and pilot-tested CHF pathways for their respective disciplines. Physical therapists participated in development of a Total Knee Replacement Pathway. The agency's first truly interdisciplinary pathway, Cerebrovascular Accident (CVA), is currently under development and includes physical therapy, occupational therapy, nursing, and social work.

Pathway Format: VNS-NW Pathways to Health©. All pathways share the same format: a) Overview with criteria for admission and list of patient-education handouts; b) pre-printed plan of care containing problem statements, expected outcomes, and nursing interventions; c) home-visit notes with pre-printed assessment cues and interventions; d) flow sheets to track outcomes achieved and document variance; and e) patient-education handouts keyed to both the plan of care and home-visit notes. An example of a pre-printed plan of care is shown in Appendix A. Problem statements rather than nursing diagnoses are used to support multi-disciplinary collaboration. Outcomes and interventions are categorized into two phases. The first phase includes the outcomes and interventions deemed essential for initial stability at home. The second phase includes outcomes and interventions focused toward ongoing self-management. Each phase contains a predetermined number of visits. Clinicians target the date by which each patient outcome should be achieved. If the outcome is not achieved by that date, the reason is documented as variance. Appendix B shows the outcome flow sheet for the Acute Wound Pathway to Health©.

Development of Generic Pathway: Outcome Based Documentation System. Throughout the pathway-development process, the effects of managed care continued to influence the VNS-NW documentation system. It became clear that streamlined documentation and formalized outcome tracking were needed for all patients. The result was design and implementation of an Outcome Based Documentation System (OBDS) for patients who are not appropriate to place on a diagnosis-specific critical pathway. This generic pathway incorporates care elements, interventions; and outcomes that are seen as common to all patients, regardless of diagnosis. The standards of "best practice" are maintained by a pre-printed outcome-focused plan of care.

Implementation: Collision of Vision and Realities

VNS-NW implemented its first critical pathways with standardized presentations by members of the development team. By experiencing the development process, team members became the critical-pathway experts at VNS-NW. Their high level of commitment was viewed as a powerful vehicle to promote pathway utilization. The combination of management and clinician team members provided a balanced perspective.

Managers selected clinician-presenters on the basis of their identified strengths and relationship to the targeted audiences, and worked together with them to individualize the standardized presentations for each branch office. Teaching strategies were determined by audience needs and characteristics. The clinician-presenters used examples from their own practice to model new information and expectations, such as the requirement to document patient response codes. They also enthusiastically volunteered to present the new patient/caregiver-education materials contained as a component of all critical pathways. As suggested by Clemmer, managers shifted from the authoritarian role into the role of coach or facilitator.[5] Collectively, they guided development of clinicians as presenters and provided consistent overall leadership.

Despite involvement of clinicians in development and introduction of the critical pathways, the RN clinical staff openly resisted their use. The previous home-visit note was primarily narrative and allowed considerable variation in documentation content. In contrast, the critical pathway home-visit note was diagnosis-specific and required focused documentation as evidence of "best practice"(Appendix C). VNS-NW was not only asking clinicians to change to a new format of documentation, but also, more importantly, was demanding they meet expectations of a new standard of practice.

Strategies to Achieve "Best Practice"

Clinician feedback, concurrent review of documentation, and analysis of outcome data provided the factual basis for ongoing evolution and redesign of critical pathways at VNS-NW. Strategies to improve clinical practice and quality of documentation resulted. Better targeting of clinician and visit resources toward realistic outcomes remains the long-term goal.

Clinician Feedback. Clinician feedback was obtained from the onset of the new documentation system. Management and RN-clinician meetings were held during the initial transition. Structured and open-ended written feedback was also solicited. Feedback was analyzed within the overall framework of defining outcomes and measuring their achievement. Some comments clearly reflected resistance to change and reluctance to being held accountable for practice. Other comments identified clinicians who understood the goals of the new system. Four categories emerged from clinician comments: a) outcome flow sheets not being updated on a timely basis; b) duplication of outcomes between the care plan and outcome flow sheet; c) confusion regarding variance codes; and d) cumbersome discharge documentation. Clinician ideas to further strengthen and streamline documentation have been carefully considered and are being integrated into the forms when appropriate to the overall pathway framework.

Concurrent Review. The management team conducted the first agency-wide concurrent review by intensively auditing compliance to the mechanical process of using OBDS. Data were benchmarked from four branch offices and aggregated for trends. Findings showed adaptation challenges to the new practice standards in three areas: identification of target visit number, completion of patient response code, and indication of outcome achievement date. The learning curve predictably varied for individual clinicians. Those with excellent critical thinking skills adapted most quickly. Within two weeks of transferring to OBDS, one of these clinicians was debating the specifics of variance assignments whereas another clinician was still overwhelmed with the mechanics of the new system. The concurrent review results were used to focus further instruction in the use of the critical pathways.

Outcome Data. Implementation of Pathways to Health© and OBDS allowed VNS-NW to begin collecting and analyzing outcome data. An early step was to count the number of visits presently required to achieve each standardized OBDS outcome. As shown in Appendix D, within 6.5 visits most patients could verbalize when to seek appropriate medical help. Fewer patients could verbalize their discharge plans within a similar time frame. Reasons for this difference are still unknown. Recognizing specific complications may be more concrete and easily mastered than understanding discharge plans. The findings may also suggest that clinical interventions emphasized immediate needs more than the planning for discharge. Because the number of visits is so limited, clinicians now must begin at the first home visit to prepare patients for discharge. Clinician education to foster this change in practice may be needed. Eventually, the agency hopes to use these data for the assignment of realistic visit targets for all standardized OBDS outcomes.

An additional step was to analyze variance data for outcomes not achieved by the clinician-assigned target date. As shown in Appendix D, two variance categories were most common for the outcomes related to seeking medical help and understanding discharge: deterioration in physiological status and psychological dysfunction. This finding may confirm the clinician assertion that patients are sicker and have more complicated home situations than they did in the past.

Another example of outcome analysis occurred with the Acute Wound Pathway to Health©. Appendix E shows data for patients admitted to the pathway since its inception. In the aggregate, all outcomes were achieved within the target visits allotted to each phase. However, the range in number of visits made varied widely. For example, a median of 3 visits was required to achieve the first Phase One outcome, "list three reportable signs/symptoms of infection or complications." Eighty-eight percent of patients or caregivers achieved the outcome within the eight visits allotted. The remaining 12% required up to 22 visits to achieve this outcome, and up to 55 visits to achieve the other Acute Wound Pathway outcomes. Fewer patients achieved the other Appendix E outcomes by the target visit. Approximately half of these patients exceeded the visit allotment only for Phase Two; the other half exceeded the allotment for both phases. Variance was greatest for the outcome, "wound healing without complications." Although this outcome was achieved within a median of ten visits, the range in visits for those patients with variance was 14 to 73.

Three variance categories were identified as trends for the outcomes shown in Appendix E: physiologic deterioration, psychological barriers, and changed physician plan. This finding is consistent with the results of the acute-wound retrospective review conducted prior to pathway design. Further analysis of the Acute Wound Pathway data will be necessary to determine whether additional resources or changed clinical practice expectations would hasten outcome achievement for outlier patients. It is also possible that the number of visits originally assigned was insufficient for the physiologically and psychologically complicated patient population.

As the diagnosis-specific Pathways to Health© and the generic OBDS have developed, there has been much evolution and cross-fertilization. Over time, criteria for placement onto diagnosis-specific critical pathways have become less rigid. The critical pathway structure has evolved to allow more individualization without losing imbedded practice standards. For example, the plan of care for the COPD pathway was designed as an algorithm, thus forcing problem choice based on assessment data. One goal of ongoing evolution is to decrease documentation redundancies and promote clinicians' systematic focus on outcomes. Another intent is to prepare VNS-NW for a computerized system.

Developing Clinicians as Resources. The clinicians who collectively make up the interdisciplinary care team are one of the most valuable resources in home health. At VNS-NW, clinicians are expected to be generalists, because they care for patients with a wide spectrum of medical diagnoses. They must simultaneously function in the roles of teacher, facilitator, and coordinator.[6] Today's clinicians experience restrictions in the number of visits authorized, increased demands for productivity, and greater accountability for managing costs. Long managers of care, clinicians are now business managers as well.

Many clinicians are concrete thinkers.[7] Now they must also think abstractly to create a strategic vision of how care can be cost effective. They must maintain visit productivity despite caring for more acutely ill patients. Clinicians are being asked to juggle heightened advocacy for patients against greater expectations for patient self-responsibility. In order to meet the health-care environment demands, clinicians must evaluate their personal and professional values and qualifications. Throughout home health there is a dichotomy between past and present expectations for practice.

The need for efficient and focused interventions, juxtaposed with a decreasing number of authorized visits, demands that today's clinicians possess the depth of knowledge and skill needed to accurately assess patient status and formulate patient problems within a short time frame. Lack of a systematic way to gather and analyze patient data may be a weak link in decision making on behalf of patients.[8] Without adequate knowledge depth, clinicians may have difficulty evaluating subtle changes in patient status and focusing on those problems most critical to positive outcomes.

The clinicians chosen to participate in developing the new VNS-NW documentation system shared knowledge and skill. Their common qualities included informal leadership among their peers, a professional approach to patient care, and collaborative interdisciplinary relationships. These clinicians were to become positive role models for "best practice." They were expected to advocate and promote use of the critical pathways and other new forms to their peers. All participating clinicians did, in fact, demonstrate a high degree of commitment throughout the development process. All also willingly participated in the implementation inservices. However, following the education and training sessions, actual use of critical pathways became a slow and cumbersome task. Normal responses to change and the change process came to the fore. Practice and care-management behaviors were being challenged, and daily operational communications were expected to become more focused and definitive. Even clinicians who participated in pathway development found themselves in the midst of the change chaos. The assumption that clinician participation would automatically foster pathway use proved untrue.

The assumption that clinicians practiced better than they documented also came into question as development proceeded. When documentation was insufficient, was knowledge also insufficient? Did generalist clinicians have enough specialized knowledge to assess key parameters and activate interventions that influenced the outcomes essential to a patient's successful self-management? These questions led to the development of knowledge tests administered in conjunction with the introduction of pathways. Tests were developed under the leadership of the agency staff-development specialist, with input from work-team members, clinicians from each office, and clinical managers. The results showed substantial knowledge gaps for some clinicians. Continuing-education classes were designed to specifically address knowledge deficits.

Yet another assumption was that an improved documentation system would automatically improve practice. We now know that "best practice" cannot be achieved by changes in documentation forms alone. Increasingly, clinician generalists may need specialty expertise, as well as their generalist breadth, in order to provide outcome-driven, high-quality, cost-effective care. Hiring and selection processes thus need to be geared toward finding the most qualified, competent human resources to promote "best practice."

Summary

Payer strategies such as limiting the visit number, prospective reimbursement, and capitation require HHAs to quantify their service delivery and resource utilization. Agencies such as VNS-NW must continually design and re-design their approaches to these payer strategies so as to achieve positive patient outcomes and remain financially viable and competitive. Evolution of outcome-based documentation through development of both diagnosis-specific and generic critical pathways has helped VNS-NW respond to environmental challenges. A documentation system that represents quality of services and quantifies results, when coupled with a clinician-development plan, will define VNS-NW "best practice" now and for the future.

References
1. L. Campbell, "Winning the Revolution," unpublished paper presented at the meeting of the Vision 2000 Seminar, Nashville, TN, 1994.
2. R.J. Ferry, "Managing Clinical Outcomes to Produce Income," *Caring* (1996): 15(6):14–17.

3. Eli's Managed Home Care, "Developing Managed Care Efficiencies Through Critical Pathways," *Managed Care Intelligence for Home Care Providers* (1995): 2:3887–3892.
4. V. Maturen and L. Van Dyck, "Using Outcome-based Critical Pathways to Improve Documentation," *Home Health Care Management and Practice.* (1996): 8(2):48–58.
5. J. Clemmer, "Pathways to Performance: An Interview With Jim Clemmer," *Joint Commission Journal of Quality Improvement* (1995): 21(4):192–200.
6. J.L. Fuzy, "Specialty Training in a Managed Care System," *Home Health Care Management and Practice* (1996): 8(3):29–35.
7. B. Goldrick, B. Gruendemann, and E. Larson, "Learning Styles and Teaching/Learning Strategy Preferences: Implications for Educating Nurses in Critical Care, the Operating Room, and Infection Control," *Heart-Lung* (1993): 22(2):176–82.
8. A.M. Jacobs and F.A. de la Cruz, "Measuring Clinical Judgment in Home Health Nursing," in C.F. Waltz and O.L. Strickland (eds.), *Measuring Clinical Skills and Professional Development in Education and Practice* (New York: Springer Publishing Company, 1988): 125–41.

APPENDIX A

Sample Plan of Care from Acute Wound Pathway to Health

Patient outcomes in the right-hand column correspond with problem and intervention statements.

VISITING NURSE SERVICES OF THE NORTHWEST

PLAN OF CARE PAGE ___ of ___

PROBLEM STATEMENT	INTERVENTION	OUTCOME	CRITICAL DATES
DATE / PROBLEM STATEMENTS:	DATE / INTERVENTIONS: SKILLED NURSING OBSERVATION (SNO) INSTRUCT AND SUPERVISE (IS) SKILLED NURSING CARE (SNC)	D/C DATE / INIT / OUTCOMES: PT/PCG WILL BE ABLE TO DEMONSTRATE OR VERBALIZE:	TARGET / MET / UNMET / INITIAL DATE
Open Wounds	SNO each visit: temp (unless <99.6 x 5 consecutive visits)		
	Wound odor, drainage, bed, surrounding skin, S/SX wound infection		
	SNO weekly BP, P, Nutrition/hydration status, wound measurements		
	IS S/S infections, complications (handout AW #1)	Reportable S/S of infection or complications	
	IS effects of secondary dx on wound healing	Impact of secondary dx on wound healing	
	IS wound care procedures (Handouts AW #2-4, 11).	Demonstrate correct wound care	
	SNC Wound Care (Specify):	At least one source for obtaining wound supplies	
		Wound healing without complications	
		Wound not healed but independent wound care	

CLINICIAN SIGNATURE   INITIALS   DATE

PATIENT NAME _____

ID# _____

APPENDIX B

Acute Wound Outcome Flow Sheet

Acute Wound Outcome Flow Sheet shows care outcomes and visit-date columns to be completed when outcomes are met. When outcomes are not achieved, the outcome number is placed in the variance section at the bottom of the form. Variance categories and codes are printed on the back of the form

VISITING NURSE SERVICES OF THE NORTHWEST

PATHWAYS TO HEALTH
ACUTE WOUND FLOW SHEET

Page ___ of ___

Patient Outcomes to be completed by the end of 13th visit (12th repeat visit). Phase I is the first 7 outcomes in the first 7 visits (repeat visit 2). Note: visit # 1 is admit visit.

If not completed by end of 8th visit for phase I and the 13th visit for phase II, record variance code and explain.

Patient/Caregiver has/is able to:	Date and initial the visit number when the outcome is completed
Visit Number E	
1. List 3 reportable s/s of infection or complications.	
2. Communicate satisfactory pain control.	
3. Verbalize understanding of using medications, effect, side effects.	
4. Verbalize understanding of nutrition/hydration for healing.	
5. Verbalize understanding of activity limitations.	
6. Demonstrate correct wound care.	
7. Adequate support systems in place.	
8. Wound healing without complications.	
9. Wound not healed; independent wound care by patient/PCG.	
10. Verbalize at least one source for obtaining wound supplies.	
11. Verbalize understanding of all medications.	
12. Verbalize impact of secondary diagnosis on wound healing.	
13. Verbalize plans for follow-up care.	
14. Manage ADLs independently or supports in place.	
15. Verbalize understanding of discharge plans.	

Outcome Number	Visit #/ Initial	Variance Code	Explanation

PATIENT NAME _____

PATIENT ID# _____

CLINICIAN SIGNATURE _____ INITIALS _____
CLINICIAN SIGNATURE _____ INITIALS _____
CLINICIAN SIGNATURE _____ INITIALS _____
CLINICIAN SIGNATURE _____ INITIALS _____

© 1994 Visiting Nurse Services of the Northwest

APPENDIX C

Home-visit Note for Acute Wound Pathway to Health

Top portion of form contains assessment cues specific to wounds. Middle section of form includes care elements, nursing interventions, and patient response codes.

VISITING NURSE SERVICES OF THE NORTHWEST

PATHWAYS TO HEALTH
ACUTE WOUND HOME VISIT NOTE

Patient Chief Complaint: _____

BP o—	BP ♀	BP ♂	AP	RP	R	T	WT	Pain Scale: (circle)
								0 1 2 3 4 5 6 7 8
								none moderate

Each Visit: Temp (unless less 99.8 consecutive visits) | Weekly: BP, pulse, respiration, nutrition/hydration status, wound measurements

ASSESSMENT DATA | **WOUND MEASUREMENTS (LENGTH, WIDTH, DEPTH) COMMENTS/LABS**

Wound odor: none q present: describe
Wound drng: none q present: describe
Wound bed: q clean q unchanged q changed/unable to visualize: describe
Surrounding skin: q clean q unchanged q changed: describe
S/S local infection: absent q present: describe
S/S systemic infection: absent q present: describe
Systems Review (CP, GI, GU, Nutrition/Hydration)

Response Codes (RC): V=verbalized D=demonstrated NR=needs reinforcement NL=no evidence of learning NA=not applicable R=refused

CARE ELEMENTS	INTERVENTIONS Assess/Instruct/Supervise Patient/Caregiver in	RC	COMMENTS
Disease Process	A Wound Care per POC q POC changed B S/S of infections, complications (Handout A) C Wound care procedures (Handouts AW #2-4) D Effects of secondary dx on wound healing		POC Change: See COO dated _____
Pain Management/ Comfort Measures	E Analgesic use, effects, side effects (Handou F Alternate comfort measures (Handout AW #		
Medication	H Knowledge of med regime, side effects (Me I Knowledge, compliance, and effectiveness o		
Nutrition/Hydration Elimination	J Nutrition/hydration for wound healing (Hand K Bowel management (Handouts AW #9, 10) L Response to diet teaching, compliance		
Mobility/ADL	M Safety precautions N Use of adaptive equipment O Activity restrictions with gradual increase as P Risks of immobility		
Psychosocial	Q Coping mechanisms		
Discharge Planning	R Support (MSW referral as indicated) S Patient/Caregiver regarding support system		
Coordination of Care	T Need for interdisciplinary, community refer		
HHA	q ORIENT q SUPERVISOR q JOINT		Patient Response to HHA POC:
Other:			Homebound q YES o NO Describe Limitations:

| TC ___ Conference
COO completed
Clinical Note complete | With:
Time: | | |

Assessment Summary/Patient Outcomes/Variances (date completed outcomes or variance)

PATIENT NAME: _____ TIME: _____ DATE: _____

ID# _____

☐ BILLABLE ☐ NONBILLABLE

© 1994 Visiting Nurse Services of the Northwest

Phase **I** Daily Visit Note q 2 q 3 q 4 q 5 q 6 q 7 q 8 (√ visit)
Additional Visit # _____
Phase **II** Daily Visit Note q 9 q 10 q 11 q 12 q 13
Additional Visit # _____

Legal CLINICIAN SIGNATURE

APPENDIX D

OBDS Average Visit and Outcome Data

Data is shown for three OBDS outcomes from Office B for May, 1996, and represents recertified and discharged patients. Using a 100% patient sample, average visit numbers, the percentage of outcomes achieved, the percent variance, and variance category trends are identified.

OBDS Outcome	Number of Patients	Average Visits	% Outcome Achieved	% Variance	Variance Category: Deteriorating Physiological Condition	Variance Category: Patient/Family Psychological Barriers
Verbalize when to seek appropriate medical help	64	6.5	80%	20%	X	X
Verbalize understanding of discharge plans	73	7.0	67%	33%	X	X
Verbalize plans for follow-up	73	7.0	67%	33%	X	X

APPENDIX E

Acute-Wound Outcome Data

Data includes the median number of visits to achieve two Phase One and two Phase Two outcomes for all patients admitted to the pathway. The percentage of outcomes achieved, percent variance, and variance category trends are identified.

Selected Acute Wound Outcomes Phase One	Number of Patients	Median Visits	% Outcome Achieved	% Variance	Variance Category: Deteriorating Physiologic Condition	Variance Category: Deteriorating Physiological Condition	Variance Category: Patient/Family Psychological Barriers
List 3 reportable s/s of infection or complications	44	3	88%	12%	X	X	
Demonstrate correct wound care	27	4	78%	22%	X	X	X
Selected Acute Wound Outcomes Phase Two							
Wound healing without complications	26	10	58%	42%	X		X
Wound not healed: independent wound care by patient/caregiver	16	8	69%	31%	X	X	X

About the Authors

Joanne Rokosky, MN, RNCS, is currently Clinical and Staff Development Specialist at Visiting Nurse Services of the Northwest. In this role she provides consultation and direct care to patients with lung disease and develops clinical resources and educational programs. She received her BSN from Pacific Lutheran University in 1968, her MN from the University of Washington in 1975. She has held ANA certification as a Clinical Specialist in Medical Surgical Nursing since 1985. Previous clinical experience includes work in medical-surgical inpatient and home health settings. She taught at the University of Washington School of Nursing and worked extensively in continuing nursing education. Among her publications are a major medical-surgical nursing textbook, which she co-authored. Honors include the American Lung Association of Washington Volunteer of the Year Award in 1993 and the King County Nurses Association Excellence in Nursing Practice Award in 1995. She is a member of the American Nurses Association, Sigma Theta Tau, and the Washington State Thoracic Society.

Cynthia Drucker, BA, CPHQ is currently Quality Improvement Manager at Visiting Nurse Services of the Northwest. In this role she coordinates the quality improvement activities and accreditation process for the agency. She received her BA in Nursing from College of Saint Scholastica in Duluth, Minnesota. She is certified as a Healthcare Quality Professional (CPHQ). Ms. Drucker worked in the home health field since 1975 and entered the quality improvement arena at VNS-NW in 1990. Previous clinical experience includes home health care casemanager, weekend nursing coordinator, and relief nursing supervisor. She is a member of the National Association of Healthcare Quality, Washington State Association of Healthcare Quality and American Nurses Association. Presently, she is co-chairperson of the Home Care Association of Washington (HCAW) Quality Improvement Committee. She was an HCAW representative member of the Washington State Health Outcomes Demonstration Project.

Joanne Ozaki-Moore, MEd, BSN, is a Patient Services Manager for the Snohomish and Skagit branch offices of Visiting Nurse Services of the Northwest. She is responsible for the daily operations of these offices. She received her BSN from the University of Washington and her Master in Adult Education Administration (MEd) from Western Washington University. She has had over twenty years of management experience in acute care, education, health maintenance organizations, and home health care. She is on the clinical faculty of the University of Washington Bothell campus. She has taught senior level courses for nursing at City University, Western Washington University and University of Guam, and has conducted workshops on quality assurance and conflict in the work place. She has co-authored a joint venture grant. She is on the advisory boards for the nursing programs at Everett Community College and Skagit Valley College and is serving as secretary for the United Way Executive Directors Association.

Chapter 4

REGISTERED NURSE USE AND PATIENT OUTCOMES IN HOME HEALTH

by Carolyn E. Adams, EdD, RN, CNAA, Associate Professor
and Robert Short, PhD, Research Associate
Washington State University, Spokane, WA

Abstract
Registered nurse (RN) time is one of the most expensive home-health agency resources. In today's market-driven environment, home-health agencies must identify where and when RN time is needed to effect positive patient outcomes. This study investigated the relationship between RN resource use and selected patient outcomes. RN resources included RN visits, RN total time, and RN mean time per visit. Three diagnosis-specific patient outcomes were measured in two groups: congestive heart failure (CHF) and diabetes mellitus (DM) patients. RN resources were related to some patient outcomes but not to others. When RN services are not related to patient outcomes, home-health agencies can investigate the possibility of using less costly providers to deliver patient services.

Introduction
One challenge in today's market-driven home-health environment is offering quality services while conserving resources. Quality is the degree to which patient care increases the probability of desired patient outcomes and reduces the probability of undesired outcomes.[1] A reputation for delivering high-quality patient care is the most important indicator of a successful home-health agency (HHA).[2] In acute-care settings, patient outcomes are tied to availability and use of registered nurses (RNs);[3] however, in home health, the relationship between RN use and patient outcomes is not well documented. Because RN time is a major home-health resource, an HHA's response to market incentives to conserve resources must encompass information on the relationship between RN time and patient outcomes.

RN Use and Patient Outcomes

A decade ago, most home-health services were paid on a fee-for-visit basis. Now, discounted fee-for-visit, capitation, and prospective payment are primary and evolving payment systems. Although distinct payment systems view HHA resources differently, in all payment systems skilled nursing care is one of the most used and costly resources. Fuzy[4] predicts that, in the future, HHAs will find themselves competing on the basis of cost of skilled-nursing visits.

The fee-for-service (FFS) payment system is cost based; HHAs are paid per visit. Traditionally, Medicare home-health services were reimbursed using this system. Under the Medicare FFS payment system, HHAs are rewarded for making more visits and maximizing costs to Medicare-determined cost limits. HHAs assume little or no financial risk for the patient in the FFS payment system. Consequently, they have few incentives to control service utilization. In fact, managing and controlling service utilization results in reduced revenues.[5]

In a FFS environment, home-health nurses averaged five to six visits daily. The average nurse visit length varied between 29 and 49 minutes.[6-9] Not surprisingly, home-health nurses paid on a fee-for-visit basis made more daily visits and shorter visits than salaried nurses.[10] In an FFS payment system, RN visit length was decreased and patient outcomes improved when RNs focused services on patient outcomes rather than on the nursing process.[9,11]

In a managed-care environment, HHAs can operate as preferred providers for health maintenance organizations (HMOs). Currently, many HHAs provide services to HMO patients at discounted fee-for-visit rates. The HHAs expect that higher patient volumes will offset discounted rates. When HHAs operate as preferred providers for HMOs, they share some of the financial risk for the patient's health. For example, visit length and care coordination time are HHA risk factors. Agencies negotiate discounted visit rates based on the average length of a visit. If HMO members require longer visits and extra care-coordination time, the HHA absorbs the excess time and costs.

Adams and associates[12] compared home-health patient outcomes and RN visit length and coordination time for Medicare patients enrolled in an HMO versus the traditional Medicare FFS program. The HHA provided services to HMO enrollees at discounted fee-for-visit rates. The number of RN visits was not significantly different for the HMO and FFS patients. Nor did RN visit length differ between the two groups. However, the HMO patients required approximately 40 minutes more nurse coordination time per care episode than the FFS patients.

Increasingly, HHAs are signing capitated contracts with HMOs. Under capitated contracts, HHAs receive a negotiated, prepaid fee for each HMO member per month. The HHA assumes the financial risk and provides all necessary home-health services to HMO members. The HMO's position is that of advocate for increased services and improved outcomes for patients.

Shaughnessy[13] compared resource utilization and patient outcomes for home-health patients in capitated and FFS systems. Almost all patients in capitated and FFS payment systems received RN visits. Home-health costs were lower in the capitated payment systems versus FFS payment systems. These findings suggest that, with capitated contracts, economic pressures result in HHAs restricting resources, including RN visits.

In 1995, the Health Care Financing Administration began testing per-episode prospective payment in home health under the National Home Health Agency Prospective Payment Demonstration.[14] Per-episode prospective payment means the home-health provider is reimbursed per patient episode of care. The reimbursement rate depends on the case-mix category of the patient. Under prospective payment, HHAs can retain savings, but they risk financial loss if a patient requires more services than the established norm. Prospective payment provides incentives for HHAs to reduce visit numbers and costs and to make the types of visits where profit margins are greatest.[15] Preliminary findings from the Prospective Payment Demonstration showed that RN visits account for about 50% of home-health visits. Among varying types of HHAs, the largest difference in episode reimbursement resulted from visit numbers rather than visit costs.[14]

Purpose of the Study

Regardless of the payment system, skilled nursing—RN care—is the most widely used and one of the most expensive home-health resources.[4] To justify use of this valuable resource, home-health providers must document the relationship between RN use and patient outcomes. The study's purpose was to describe the relationship between nurse resources used and patient outcomes in an HHA.

Methods

Design.
A descriptive correlational research design was used in the study. This study was part of a larger investigation on patient outcomes and resource use.[9, 11-12]

Setting.
The setting was a hospital-based HHA. The RN staff made about 30,000 visits annually. Agency services were reimbursed under both FFS and HMO discounted fee-for-visit payment systems.

Sample and sampling.

A convenience sample of 127 patients was used. Congestive heart failure (CHF) was the primary diagnosis of 62 patients, and diabetes mellitus (DM) the primary diagnosis of 65 patients. The sample included patients who were discharged from the HHA to home. Patients discharged to an inpatient facility or who died were not included. All patients verbalized willingness to participate in the home-health plan of care.

Study Variables.

The study variables were RN resource-utilization measures and patient-outcome indicators. Three resource-utilization measures were used: a) number of RN visits; b) total number of RN minutes used to care for a patient (hereafter termed "RN total minutes"); and c) average length of a RN patient visit (hereafter termed "RN mean minutes"). Number of RN visits was the number of billed visits the nurse made to the patient. RN total minutes was the total amount of time RNs used caring for the patient during the care episode. Care coordination time—telephoning, conferencing, charting—was not included in the total time. RN mean minutes was the RN total minutes divided by the number of RN visits to a patient.

For the CHF patient group, the following outcome indicators were assessed: a) uses activity pacing to manage dyspnea; b) weight stabilized for three weeks; and c) demonstrates how to take radial pulse. For the DM patient group, the outcome indicators were: a) demonstrates correct blood-glucose monitoring technique; b) achieves blood-glucose level in range prescribed by physician; and c) verbalizes signs and symptoms of hypoglycemia. The outcome indicators were expected patient outcomes listed on standardized care plans. In addition, the HHA quality-improvement committee members identified the outcomes as important indicators of home-health quality for the populations studied.

Procedure.

As patients were discharged, patient and agency records were reviewed and information extracted. Number of nurse visits was counted on the agency computerized billing form. Total RN nurse time was tabulated from computerized summaries of the nurses' daily itineraries. On the itineraries, nurses recorded the time they left their vehicle to enter a patient's home and the time they returned to the vehicle. The length of each RN patient visit was summed to obtain the RN total time for each patient.

Outcome-indicator data were collected from patient records and nurse daily-visit records. If any record showed that the outcome was achieved, the item was scored as "outcome achieved." If records revealed the outcome was not achieved or no documentation was present, the item was scored as "outcome not achieved." Agency staff knew the patients were being studied. They did not know the outcome indicators studied nor that resource-utilization data were collected.

Results

The average age of the CHF sample was 81.5 years (SD=8.4 years). For the DM patients, the average age was 71.4 years (SD=11.6 years). Selected characteristics of the CHF and DM samples are in Table 1. The high percent of Caucasians in the sample reflects the region's racial homogeneity. On the characteristic "mobility," common assistive devices used were canes and walkers.

Table 1
Characteristics of the CHF and DM Patients on Admission

Characteristics	CHF (n=62) f	%	DM (n=65) f	%
Gender				
Female	41	66%	43	66%
Male	21	34%	22	34%
Race				
Caucasian	61	98%	59	91%
Black	1	2%	3	4.6%
Asian	0	0%	3	4.6%
Marital Status				
Married	19	31%	32	49%
Widowed	35	56%	24	37%
Single	8	13%	9	14%
Caregiver Available				
Yes	38	61%	42	65%
No	24	39%	23	35%
Manages Care				
Self	16	26%	24	37%
Caregiver Assists	36	58%	33	51%
Caregiver Provides	10	16%	8	12%
Mobility				
Walks Alone	28	45%	36	55%
Uses Assistive Device	29	47%	23	35%
Wheelchair/Bedbound	5	8%	6	9%

Descriptive statistics were calculated for the three resource-utilization measures—RN visits, RN total minutes, and RN mean minutes—for both the CHF and DM groups (Table 2). For the resource utilization measures, the median was a better indicator of central tendency than the mean because distributions were asymmetrical. In the CHF group, the median patient received eight visits, and required 342.5 RN total minutes; each RN visit averaged 44.3 minutes. In the DM group, the median patient received eight visits, and required 336.0 total minutes of RN care; each RN visit lasted an average of 44.2 minutes.

Table 2
Descriptive Statistics of RN Visits, RN Total Minutes, and RN Mean Minutes for the CHF (n=62) and DM (n=65) Patients

Variable	Mean (SD)	Median	Minimum	Maximum
CHF Patients				
# Visits	12.6 (2.3)	8.0	1.0	176.0
Total Minutes	586.3 (989.7)	342.5	66.0	7,791.0
Mean Minutes	53.8 (37.9)	44.3	26.2	245.0
DM Patients				
# Visits	13.0 (16.4)	8.0	1.0	115.0
Total Minutes	555.8 (788.7)	336.0	101.0	5,944.0
Mean Minutes	48.0 (16.6)	44.2	7.6	115.0

For each outcome indicator, the frequency and percentage of patients who achieved and did not achieve the outcomes were calculated (Table 3). Outcome indicators not applicable for a patient were not included in the calculations. For example, if blood-glucose monitoring was not ordered, the patient was not included in the tabulation of patients who achieved or did not achieve the blood glucose monitoring.

Table 3
Frequency and Percent of Patients Who Achieved and Did Not Achieve Each Outcome

Outcome	Achieved f*	%	Not Achieved f*	%
CHF Patients (n=62)				
Activity Pacing	35	56%	27	44%
Radial Pulse	12	19%	50	81%
Stable Weight	21	38%	34	62%
DM Patients (n=65)				
Hypoglycemia Knowledge	34	53%	30	47%
Blood-Glucose Level	45	69%	20	31%
Blood-Glucose Monitoring	62	97%	2	3%

*Because outcomes were not applicable to all patients, some outcome frequencies do not sum to the diagnosis sample sizes.

When the three resource-utilization measures were plotted on histograms, all showed positively skewed distributions. Consequently, raw scores were recoded into three categories forming low, moderate, and high levels for each resource utilization measure (Table 4).

Table 4
Resource Use Measures Recoded Into Low, Medium, and High Levels for CHF (n=62) and DM (n=65) Patients

Resource Use	Low Range	%	Moderate Range	%	High Range	%
CHF Patients						
# Visits	1—5	30%	6—10	38%	11—176	32%
Total Min.	66—300	37%	300.1—480	29%	80.1—7791	34%
Mean Min.	26—40	34%	40.1—50	32%	50.1—245	34%
DM Patients						
# Visits	1—5	30%	6—10	33%	11—115	37%
Total Min.	101—300	38%	300.1—480	33%	480.1—5,944	29%
Mean Min.	7.6—40	32%	40.1—50	28%	50.1—115	40%

Chi-square analyses were completed to compare the RN resource-utilization measures for patients who achieved or did not achieve each outcome indicator (Table 5). The relationship between the outcome indicator "uses activity pacing to manage dyspnea" and both RN visit number and RN total minutes were statistically significant (p<.05).

Table 5
Chi-square Summary Assessing Relationship Between Resource Utilization Measures and Patient Outcomes

Outcome	# Visits	Chi-square values* Total Min.	Mean Min.
CHF Patients (n=62)			
Activity Pacing	18.4302†	9.6881†	3.0761
Stable Weight	4.8887	1.2301	.1542
DM Patients (n=65)			
Hypoglycemia Knowledge	13.9773†	5.1800‡	8.1485†
Blood-Glucose Level	.4514	1.3890	.3038

*df=2, †p<.05, ‡p=.07

Overall, patients with more RN visits and greater RN total time achieved the outcome more often. Of the patients who received moderate and high visit numbers, 74% achieved the desired outcome, while 26% did not. For patients who received low visit numbers, only 16% achieved the outcome, while 84% did not. Similarly, results were found for RN total minutes. Of the patients who received moderate and high RN total minutes, 73% achieved the desired outcome. This contrasted with patients who received low RN total minutes; only 35% of these patients achieved the outcome.

The chi-square value between "verbalizes signs and symptoms of hypoglycemia" and visit number was significant ($p<.05$). Of the patients who received a moderate or high number of visits, 74% achieved the outcome. Only 16% of patients who received a low number of visits achieved the outcome. Although not statistically significant ($p=.07$), the same relationship was found for RN total minutes. While 62% of patients who received a moderate or high amount of RN total minutes achieved the outcome, 38% of patients receiving low amounts of RN total minutes achieved the outcome.

The chi-square value between "verbalizes signs and symptoms of hypoglycemia" and RN mean minutes was significant ($p<.05$). However, only 24% of patients who received longer (high) RN mean minutes achieved the outcome. Unexpectedly 72% of patients who received the shorter visits (low and moderate) achieved the outcome.

The chi-square values between each resource utilization measure and the outcomes "weight stabilized for three weeks" and "achieves blood-glucose level in prescribed range" were not statistically significant ($p>.05$). When the chi-square analyses were completed between the resource-utilization measures and the outcomes "demonstrates correct blood-glucose monitoring technique" and "demonstrates how to take radial pulse," cell frequencies were so small that the chi-squares were invalid. These chi-square values are not reported.

Discussion and Implications

RN resource use and patient outcomes were measured to determine how RN resource use was related to patient achievement of selected outcome measures. RN resource utilization measures were RN visit number, RN total minutes, and RN mean minutes. Three diagnosis-specific outcomes were measured for CHF and DM patients. For two outcome indicators, use of more RN resources resulted in more patients achieving the outcomes. The outcome indicators were "uses activity pacing to manage dyspnea" for the CHF group and "verbalizes signs and symptoms of hypoglycemia" for the DM group. Two outcome indicators—"weight stabilized for three weeks" and "achieves blood-glucose level in prescribed range"—were not significantly related to RN resource use. Statistically valid chi-squares could not be calculated between the resource use measures and the outcomes "demonstrates correct blood-glucose monitoring technique" and "demonstrates how to take a radial pulse."

The findings support and extend those of Shaughnessy and associates.[13] Shaughnessy found that, in comparison to home-health patients who received fewer services, patients who received more agency services had better outcomes. Shaughnessy's findings were descriptive; the relationship between agency services and patient outcomes was not statistically tested. The present study provides statistical documentation of a significant relationship between resource use and patient outcomes: When more RN resources were used, more patients achieved the outcomes.

Outcome selection is an important factor when studying the relationship between resource utilization and patient outcomes. For the outcome "demonstrates correct blood-glucose monitoring technique" almost all patients (97%) achieved the outcome; and for "demonstrates how to take a radial pulse," few (24%) achieved the outcome. The chi-square cell frequencies were not large enough to complete chi-square analyses between levels of RN resource use and either outcome. When relating a patient outcome to resource utilization, the outcome must vary sufficiently in the sample to allow valid statistical tests. Outcomes which almost all patients achieve or which almost no patients achieve are not useful variables for estimating the relationship between resource utilization and patient outcomes.

RN resource use was related to some patient outcomes but not to others. For example, although RN time was significantly related to "uses activity pacing to manage dyspnea" and "verbalizes signs and symptoms of hypoglycemia," RN time was not significantly related to "weight stabilized for three weeks" and "achieves blood-glucose level in prescribed range." RN time is an expensive resource and must be used wisely. HHAs should identify which patient outcomes are influenced by RN time. RNs can be used to provide patient services related to these outcomes. However, when patient outcomes are not influenced by RN time, HHAs can determine if less costly resources, e.g., licensed vocational nurses or nursing assistants, can provide patient services.

Overall, more DM patients than CHF patients achieved the outcomes. By discharge, 97% of the DM group demonstrated blood-glucose monitoring, 69% achieved blood-glucose levels in prescribed ranges, and 53% verbalized signs and symptoms of hypoglycemia. In contrast, in the CHF group, only 56% used activity pacing to manage dyspnea, 38% achieved a stable weight, and 19% were able to take a radial pulse. The average age of the DM group was 71.4 years, while the average age of the CHF group was 81.5 years. Very likely, age is a case-mix factor that must be considered when relating resource utilization to patient outcomes.

For the outcome indicator "verbalizes signs and symptoms of hypoglycemia," 72% of patients who averaged shorter (low and moderate RN mean time) visits achieved the outcome. Only 24% of patients who averaged longer (high) RN mean minutes achieved the outcome. These findings may be related to earlier research[9] showing an inverse relationship between RN visit length and improved outcomes when RNs focused on patient outcomes rather than the nursing process. Alternatively, the apparent association between RN mean time and "verbalizes signs and symptoms of hypoglycemia" may be a mathematical artifact. Because RN visit number (with a high association with the outcome) was divided into RN total minutes (with a non-significant association with the outcome), an apparent negative relationship was produced between RN mean minutes and "verbalizes signs and symptoms of hypoglycemia."

Limitations and Future Studies

Generalization of the study results is limited by the methods used to collect the data. A convenience sample was used. Future investigations should use random sampling procedures to enhance generalization of results. Further, the setting was a not-for-profit, hospital-based HHA. Resources are used differently by for-profit versus not-for-profit, freestanding versus hospital-based, and rural versus urban HHAs.[14] The relationship between RN resource use and patient outcomes must be explored in other types of HHAs.

The outcome indicators were developed by the investigators and staff of the study HHA. The indicators were validated by expert opinion of agency nurses and nursing textbooks. No inter-rater reliability was used to identify if nurses documented achievement or non-achievement of the indicators in the same way. To more fully understand the relationship between RN resource use and patient outcomes, validated and reliable outcome measures are needed. After the current study was started, the Outcome Assessment and Information Set (OASIS) developed for the National Medicare Quality Assurance and Improvement Demonstration was published.[16] OASIS provides standardized patient-outcomes measures. In the future, researchers should consider using items from OASIS in studies describing resource use and patient outcomes.

References
1. Joint Commission on Accreditation of Healthcare Organizations, *1995 Accreditation Manual for Home Care,* Volume I, *Standards* (Oakbrook, IL: JCAHO, 1995).
2. P.A. Cloonan and B.M. Brodie, "Home Healthcare Agencies: What Constitutes Success," *Nursing Economics* (1993): 11(1):29—33.
3. American Nurses Association, *Nursing Care Report Card for Acute Care* (Washington, DC: ANA, 1995).
4. J.L. Fuzy, "Specialty Training in a Managed Care System," *Home Health Care Management and Practice* (1996): 8(3):29—35.

5. K.C. Jones, "Managed Care: The Coming Revolution in Home Health Care," *Journal of Home Health Care Practice* (1994): 6(2):1—11.
6. C.S. Hedtcke, I. MacQueen, and A. Carr, "How do Home Health Nurses Spend Their Time?" *Journal of Nursing Administration* (1992): 22(1):18—22.
7. M.G. Trisolini, C.P. Parks, S.B. Cashman, and S.M. Payne, "Resource Utilization in Home Health Care: Results of a Prospective Study," *Home Health Care Services Quarterly* (1994): 15(1):19—39.
8. J.L. Helberg, "Resource Utilization in Home Care: Methods and Issues," *Nursing & Health Care* (1990): 11(9):464—68.
9. C.E. Adams and N. Biggerstaff, "Reduced Resource Utilization Through Standardized Outcome-focused Care Plans," *Journal of Nursing Administration* (1995): 25(10):43—50.
10. Y. Luque and K. Crocket, "Pay-per-visit for Staff: Saving Money Without Sacrificing Quality of Care," *Caring* (1990): 9(2):16—18, 20.
11. C.E. Adams and M. Wilson, "Enhanced Quality Through Outcome-focused Standardized Care Plans," *Journal of Nursing Administration* (1995): 25(9):27—34.
12. C.E. Adams, R. Usher, and S. Kramer, "Home Health Nurse Patient Care and Coordination Time: Health Maintenance Organization Versus Fee-for-Service," *Journal of Nursing Administration* (1997): 27(3): in press.
13. P.W. Shaughnessy, R.E. Schlenker, and D.F. Hittle, *A Study of Home Health Care Quality and Cost Under Capitated and Fee-for-Service Payment Systems* (Denver: Center for Health Policy Research, 1994).
14. H.B. Goldberg and R.J. Schmitz, "Contemplating Home Health PPS: Current Patterns of Medicare Service Use," *Health Care Financing Review* (1994): 16(1):109—30.
15. B.R. Phillips, R.S. Brown, C.E. Bishop, A.C. Klein, G.A. Ritter, J.L. Schore, K.C. Skwara, and C.V. Thornton, "Do Preset Per Visit Payment Rates Affect Home Health Agency Behavior?" *Health Care Financing Review* (1994): 16(1):91—107.
16. P.W. Shaughnessy and K.S. Crisler, *Outcome-Based Quality Improvement: A Manual for Home Care Agencies on How to Use Outcomes* (Washington, DC: National Association for Home Care, 1995).

About the Authors

Carolyn E. Adams, EdD, RN, CNAA is Associate Professor at the College of Nursing, Washington State University. Her specialty is organizational systems and leadership. Dr. Adams operates as an intrapreneur within the college of nursing offering consultation and research in home health outcomes and resource optimization. Dr. Adams is a well-published author and international consultant in home health outcomes. Currently, Dr. Adams is primary investigator in the Washington State Home Health Outcomes Standards Demonstration.

Robert Short, PhD is presently a member of the core staff at the Washington Institute for Mental Illness Research and Training at Washington State University at Spokane. Dr. Short has published over 30 articles in a variety of peer reviewed books and journals, and has contributed to several successful major federal research grants. As well, Dr. Short does statistical consulting with staff from regional hospitals and colleges, including the research nursing faculty at the Intercollegiate Center for Nursing Education in Spokane.

Chapter 5

UTILIZING PATIENT SATISFACTION TO MEET THE CHALLENGES OF MANAGED HEALTH CARE

by Nancy Yezzi Moran, MS, RN, *Consultant*
and Mary P. Malone, MS, JD, CHE, *Vice President,
Corporate Development, Press, Ganey Associates, Inc.*

Abstract
As the managed-care, outcomes, and accountability movements extend their reach to home-care providers, patient-satisfaction data will assume an even greater role. Measuring, monitoring, and using patient-satisfaction information will be a critical success factor for agency executives. This article examines reasons why patient satisfaction will assume this role, and factors home-care providers should consider when implementing patient-satisfaction programs.

The discussion will include a review of the patient-satisfaction measurement process in home care, and survey design techniques and the implementation process. Emphasis is placed on utilizing patient-satisfaction survey data as an external reference point for comparing agency performance in a national database comprised of home-care agencies. The relationship between patient-satisfaction data and quality-improvement programs will be discussed, as well as the importance of linking patient-satisfaction data to clinical and financial outcomes.

Introduction
In 1993, the United States spent more than $850 billion—14% of the gross national product—on health care. If the current rate of spending continues, this figure is estimated to exceed one trillion dollars in 1997.[1] In an effort to reduce the costs of the patient-care delivery system, payers and providers have expanded the utilization of home health-care services. Annual home-care expenditures for 1996 were expected to exceed $36 billion.[2]

As the point of service shifts to the home setting, many factors will need to be assessed in order to evaluate the success of this cost-containment strategy. The accountability and outcomes revolutions affect home care in this regard. Payers, employers, managed-care plans, other providers, and accrediting agencies are demanding information regarding outcomes. Outcomes generally fall into four categories: cost/financial, clinical, functional status, and patient satisfaction. To be accountable to these external organizations, a home-care agency must be able to demonstrate successful outcomes in all four areas. Managed-care initiatives will cause patient satisfaction to be a critical success factor for home-care agencies, since few **payers** are likely to contract with a home-care agency that dissatisfies its patients.

Patient Satisfaction as a Critical Success Factor
Home-care administrators recognize the need to query patients about the services the agency provides. Home-care executives can list many factors that contribute to the emphasis on customer service/patient satisfaction.

1. Providing high-quality service is part of the mission statement of most agencies, and requires satisfying patients and their families.
2. Patient satisfaction relates to the bottom-line financial results of an agency.
3. The ability to show high levels of patient satisfaction to payers, employers, providers, and managed-care organizations can help an agency demonstrate successful outcomes.
4. Satisfying patients contributes to the quality of their lives and can help increase compliance with medical regimes.
5. Satisfied patients are important for word-of-mouth referrals and for helping the external image of an agency.
6. Satisfied patients can help increase employee satisfaction, and positively influence recruitment and retention.
7. Satisfying patients is more cost effective than responding to complaints.
8. Quality-improvement initiatives require data about patient satisfaction.

In the inpatient setting, systematic approaches to measuring patient satisfaction were not available until about a dozen years ago. Today, as outcomes measurement and quality-improvement initiatives have become important management strategies, nearly all hospital systems have adopted strategic initiatives for measuring, monitoring, and improving patient satisfaction.

Systematic measurement of home-care patient satisfaction is still in its infancy. Home-care executives are just beginning to recognize the paramount importance of patient-satisfaction information, particularly as it relates to strategic competitive advantage and to providing information to external audiences. The movement toward more systematic measurement is likely to occur quickly as integration between home-care providers and hospitals continues.

As managed-care initiatives place increasing pressure on home-care providers, and the home-care industry moves toward implementing quality-improvement programs, managers will be asked to define their customers and to focus, increasingly, on customer perceptions. Total quality management and continuous quality improvement (TQM/CQI) programs place a high value on collecting and analyzing data regarding customer satisfaction. To effectively participate in quality-improvement initiatives, home-care agencies must have accurate, systematic approaches to measuring patient satisfaction. The successful home-care agency cannot delay in implementing programs for measuring, monitoring, and improving patient satisfaction; the data are too important to occupy a subsidiary position in an agency's strategic plan. Sufficient resources must be allocated to measure and to implement quality-improvement activities based upon the results.

Traditional Approaches to Home-Care Surveys
Historically, agencies utilized in-house surveys developed by agency personnel. These surveys have often been poorly designed. Pontin and Webb note that the main problems associated with gauging patient satisfaction often relate to acceptable and valid survey tools.[3]

Traditionally, surveys were administered sporadically, and the quality of the results reported varied considerably. Often, the in-house survey and reports were designed not for quality improvement, but to appease board members, owners, and management, or to justify the status quo. Many home-care providers report results such as 95% satisfied, often by collapsing response scales (see the appendix). These results are not helpful to the quality initiatives, since they support an erroneous perception that nearly all patient needs are being met and service delivery does not need to improve.

Westra, et. al., report that survey design needs to evaluate client expectations and perceptions of the care received.[4] Specifically, patient expectations are related to the type of care provided, the number and types of care providers, the kinds of interactions encountered, and the setting in which the care was provided. Domains of these evaluations include

- art of care (interpersonal relationships);
- technical care;
- financial aspects;
- access and convenience;
- physical environment;
- availability of care;
- interpersonal educational relationship;
- continuity of care and efficacy; and
- overall satisfaction.[5–7]

66   Nancy Yezzi Moran, Mary P. Malone

Implementing Patient Surveys: A New Approach
Given the strategic importance of patient satisfaction, it is likely to attract the interest of home-care executives, particularly as they respond to the data requirements of their external audiences. Quality experts agree that the most crucial variable in successful implementation of a customer-satisfaction monitoring program is senior management's commitment to the process. Once management has lent its support to the goals and objectives of customer-satisfaction monitoring, the process can proceed.

Listed below are some factors to consider when implementing or reviewing a patient satisfaction monitoring system.

1. What type of survey—mail, telephone, or interview—is appropriate, given the type of data the agency is seeking? Is anonymity an important consideration, so that patients feel free to give honest answers without fear of reprisals? This might dictate written surveys.[8,9]

2. Who will be surveyed? Each patient or a sample of patients? How will the sample be drawn? How will the agency address issues of incapable or incompetent patients? Many home-care providers are still developing information systems that will support the process. How often should the survey be conducted? Is the desired information something that should be monitored at least quarterly? Can the survey be conducted on an ongoing basis for a sample of newer, older, and continuing patients?

3. What type of questions should be asked, and what response framework should be used? Do the questions make sense—are they relevant to the patient's overall evaluation of the home-care experience? Questions must reflect issues of importance to patients, not administrators, and should be derived from patients' concerns. This is critical, because a poorly designed survey generates suspect data.

4. How long should the survey be? How will the survey balance a desire to obtain very specific data through asking many questions and the negative impact that a longer survey can have on response rates?

5. Which personal data—age, gender, principal diagnosis, general health status—should be included?. How will that information be used in processing that data? Will asking these types of questions affect the willingness of the patients to respond, especially those who remain under the care of the agency?

6. Is the wording of the questions clear and unbiased? Which statistical tests will be used to judge the validity and reliability of the survey? When the data is tabulated, will it produce meaningful and actionable results?

7. How often should the results be tabulated and distributed? How should the results be presented? What statistics will be most useful? Will the format be usable by upper management, supervisory staff, and employees? How should written comments be handled?
8. How will the results be acted upon? Who will receive them? How will the results be communicated to all employees? What mechanisms will be utilized to reward improvements in the scores?
9. What resources will a monitoring program require? Is management willing to commit the resources needed to effectively perform the process? What are the guarantees that the results will be taken seriously and acted upon?
10. How will the results be communicated to external audiences such as payers, employers, managed-care plans, provider networks, and others?

One Approach to Survey Development
Irwin Press, PhD, and Rodney Ganey, PhD, co-founders of Press, Ganey Associates, Inc., have measured patient satisfaction with health-care experiences since 1985. In 1993, the firm developed a tool to monitor quality in the home-health field. The firm's expertise lies in developing tested and reliable satisfaction surveys, comprehensive management reports, and national, comparative databases.

The development of the firm's home-care satisfaction measurement tool began by conducting interviews and focus groups with home-care patients, their families, and home-care executives. The survey was designed to elicit honest appraisals, maximize returns, and promote written comments pertaining to the home-care experience. The development process concluded with testing at 12 sites around the country. The test sites included both hospital-based home-health agencies and freestanding home-health agencies. The final version of the survey consists of a set of core (or standard) questions which evaluate the home-care patient's experiences with nurses and home-care aides, arranging care, and dealing with the office. While the "core" questions cover the range of topics and issues that will most likely be of importance to a patient, the agencies retain the flexibility to tailor the survey to their needs (including adding customized questions).

As of early 1997, nearly 200 home-care providers are under contract to utilize the core survey and to receive national comparative (benchmarking data) from the firm. Agencies have confidence that surveys will produce statistically valid and reliable data. The survey and the report have enabled home-health agencies nationwide to evaluate the quality of care provided to patients who are quite aware of what matters to them. In addition, the firm provides analysis of the written comments. The comments provided by patients on the surveys are categorized by positive, negative, and mixed ratings. While the core questions provide the uniformity necessary to gather data for benchmarking, the written comments can provide an agency with information that pertains quite specifically to an experience patients may have had while receiving care.

A Note About Methodology
There are three main approaches for gathering patient-satisfaction data: written surveys, telephone surveys, and personal interviews. The goal for researchers is to match the data-gathering technique to the situation. Researchers at Press, Ganey have weighed the relative strengths and weaknesses of each method, and have elected to use a written (mail) methodology for collecting patient-satisfaction data. Several researchers, including Ware and Press and Hall, have noted that patients are reluctant to criticize those who have provided health care to them for fear of retaliation. With telephone surveying, patients can lose the ability to speak anonymously of disruptions or disappointments in their care. Without the safety of anonymity, patients may be inclined to skew their responses toward the positive, and, as a result, problem areas may remain hidden. This form of bias is referred to as "acquiescence bias," and it can lessen the validity of an agency's survey data. For these reasons, Press, Ganey researchers support written (mail) surveys as the least intrusive to client privacy and for generating the least biased response.

Mailing surveys to patients also gives the patient's family the opportunity to provide input into the survey responses. Some health-care providers may be concerned with the family's participation in the completion of the survey. However, the family often provides input at all stages of a patient's care. The completed questionnaire can provide an indication of how the patient and his/her family feel about the care received, as well as what their follow-up to service will be—for example, recommend changes to the agency, complain to the physician or managed-care organization, or seek legal advice.

Analysis of the National Database
Recently, researchers at Press, Ganey compiled data based upon the results of 14,324 surveys from 51 home-care agencies. A standard survey question, "likelihood of recommending the home-care agency," was correlated with the responses to the other standard survey questions. The top ten issues, based upon the magnitude of the correlation coefficients, are reported below.

1. Staff concern to keep family informed about treatment, condition, and progress
2. How well the agency handled emergencies

3. Nurse's sensitivity to the personal difficulties and inconveniences caused by your health problem
4. How well the nurse teaches you to care for yourself
5. Technical skill of the nurse
6. Nurse's attention to your own ideas about your care
7. Family involvement in planning home-health services
8. How well agency handles request to change nurse/aide
9. How well initial plan of health care or treatment met your needs
10. Nurse's concern for your comfort while treating you

Home-care agencies should note that these are the questions that are most highly correlated with likelihood of recommending the agency. These areas are important ones, upon which the industry should focus limited resources. Nearly all of them involve interpersonal interactions between the patient and the caregiver. Interestingly, none of the top issues involve billing or cost concerns.

Additional Advantages of Benchmarking Data
Even when a home-care agency performs ongoing patient-satisfaction monitoring, one additional consideration remains. An agency which performs its own patient-satisfaction monitoring, using an internally developed and internally analyzed survey, lacks an external reference point.

While the agency with an internal system is capable of monitoring trends within its own departments (and it could produce more sophisticated statistics such as correlation coefficients based upon its own data), it lacks the ability to judge whether the standards or goals it is setting are realistic, given certain characteristics (such as community size/location, Medicare certification, annual visit volume, and the types of services provided) that may have an overall affect on its customers' perceptions.

There are several reasons for using an external reference point. If an agency uses its internal survey and receives a score of 85.1 for "how well costs were explained" and a score of 87.2 for "nurse's concern for your comfort while treating you" (see the appendix for a note about calculating scores), the agency manager is likely to commend the nurse for a job well done and demand improvements from the billing manager. However, external comparisons might show that, nationwide the score of 85.1 is the highest ever achieved in billing explanations, and 87.2 is the lowest ever achieved on the issue of concern for comfort shown by a nurse.

Without comparative data, the home-care manager has made the wrong decisions, and is wasting resources to try to improve an area that is doing relatively well (cost explanations), while an area in need of improvement (concern for comfort shown by nurse) is receiving undeserved recognition. Furthermore, analysis of correlation coefficients might suggest that satisfaction with the concern of the nurse is more highly associated with overall satisfaction than billing explanations. While explanations about cost are important, and each department should participate in improvement activities to achieve the highest levels of satisfaction, the agency would be better off spending more effort enhancing the nurses' ability to provide for the patients' comfort. Ignoring this type of information might endanger the long-term viability of the agency, since overall patient satisfaction is a critical success factor, and focusing on areas that have little impact on patient satisfaction wastes valuable resources.

Home-care agency executives should take benchmarking data into account when setting quality-improvement goals. It simply may be unrealistic to expect huge increases in patient-satisfaction scores for certain areas, such as billing; more modest goals might be appropriate. Without an external reference point, goals may be set—and incentive programs established—which the agency has no chance of achieving. Unrealistic goals can be demoralizing for everyone.

Home-care agencies might also be interested in the opportunity to develop a hand-picked database, or "peer group." Selected for particular characteristics, the agencies in a peer group will most often share a certain feature, e.g., region, agency size, types of services. The peer-group comparison allows the agency to further compare their scores and identify any noteworthy relationships between their agency and others within their hand-picked database.

The process utilized by the JCAHO to review home-health agencies for accreditation requires agencies to benchmark information from similar agencies. Other national organizations that oversee the evaluation of home-health agencies expect comparisons of data or information which will effectively indicate the level of quality of the services provided. Additionally, those accrediting organizations implement changes based on the results of patient-satisfaction data.

Linking Patient Satisfaction Data to Clinical/Financial Data
What measures does the home-health agency take to effectively communicate its quality, as evidenced by their patient-satisfaction scores, when working with managed-care companies? An important feature of the survey process can be the ability to precode patient-satisfaction surveys. Precoding generally means attaching a label containing either a unique patient identifier or several important data elements about the patient. These data elements might include principal diagnosis, payer, physician, case manager, home-care aide, and other demographic information specific to the patient. Of course, patients should be

assured that the information will not be used to identify them, and that the survey can still be completed anonymously.

By including a precoded label on the survey (or the unique patient identifier) an agency will receive many benefits. In addition to standard analysis of the overall scores for the questions contained on the survey (and benchmarks if the agency is using a standard survey), the agency will also have the ability to break down that information as it pertains to certain areas that have been precoded. Reports can be provided in areas such as patient satisfaction by a patient's length of stay on service, insurance type/payer, employer, state of health, primary diagnosis code, referral source, and demographic information. This additional "drill-down" analysis can be extremely helpful in identifying areas that are exemplary and those in need of improvement. Without identification of those areas in need of improvement, changes will less likely be made in the agency's CQI plan, and, consequently, in the agency's scores.

Furthermore, an agency that precodes its surveys using a unique patient identifier can receive patient survey results in a data file that can be linked back to other computerized clinical/financial information, providing, of course, that the unique patient identifier is common to both files. This permits even more sophisticated data analysis.

Responding to Managed Care and External Demands for Quality
Equipped with reliable patient-satisfaction data, the agency is prepared to identify opportunities for improvement and then implement plans for change. How exactly is quality service measured? Shaughnessy reports that agencies are developing CQI plans which include three specific types of quality measures: structure, process, and outcome.[10] CQI programs have been developed with specific standards for each type of treatment or service provided by agency personnel. Agencies have put into place policies and procedures requiring documentation for personnel qualifications, therapy, and equipment protocols to fulfill their quest to define quality.

How will quality be defined in the future? An increasing array of health-care purchasers will demand outcome indicators and proof of quality provided by the home-health agency. According to Allred, et. al., establishing linkages among individuals and institutions in order to establish a "value driven pattern of care" is the goal of managed care.[11] A "value driven delivery system" strives to be cost effective, not only to lower costs, but also to ensure that consumers receive the most effective care for the least amount of money.

The individual patient is no longer considered the typical customer. Rather, health maintenance organizations, physician provider organizations, employer coalitions, and other purchasers buy health care on behalf of the customers and employees. Managed care typically implies some type of arrangement whereby a network of providers agrees to deliver a predetermined package of health-care services to a defined population for a negotiated payment.

Agencies are prepared to identify opportunities for improvement and implement plans for change when equipped with statistically valid patient-satisfaction data. Improving quality takes a commitment from everyone involved, from the chief executive officer to those employees who are in contact with the patients daily.

Utilizing patient-satisfaction data is a vital component in meeting the challenges of the managed health-care industry. Many freestanding home-health agencies and those with integrated delivery systems have taken the lead from education and developed a performance "report card" to effectively inform consumers and other external audiences about the quality of their service. Ultimately, the report card serves as the primary marketing strategy when negotiating managed-care contracts.

One Application of Data in Quality-Improvement and Incentive Programs
Many agencies have developed employee incentive programs. With a little creativity, non-cash incentives can provide just as much motivation without incurring additional expense. In 1995, the Visiting Nurse Health System (VNHS) in Atlanta, Georgia, identified a need to benchmark satisfaction data and adopted the Press, Ganey home health-care survey.

Having familiarity in measuring patient satisfaction, VNHS executives identified early on how to utilize their patient-satisfaction scores to improve their services and establish incentive programs. Working with their home-health aide department, the company identified a desire to improve this service within the organization. Changes were made in the agency dress code and time was spent briefing aides on professional conduct. By the end of the next quarter, when the next report was received, administration saw an increase in both patient-satisfaction scores and morale among the home-health aides.

In 1996, VNHS looked more closely at their scores because they identified their customers as patients, physicians, and, most definitely, the payers or managed-care organizations. Through contract negotiations, they realized a need to illustrate in detail how satisfied patients are with the VNHS.

Looking Into the Future
In the evolving health-care environment of managed-care contracts, government regulations, and the formation of health-care networks and alliances, it is certain that home health care must focus on the three fundamental elements: cost, quality, and outcomes. As outcomes-satisfaction data become more important, home-care executives will seek to improve the process by which patient-satisfaction data is gathered and reported. One approach, common in

other service industries, is to contract with survey measurement firms. While the services these firms provide vary, they share several common features. The firms use surveys that are well researched, methodologically sound, and focused on issues important to patients. Many use standard surveys that allow the results to be benchmarked; this means that satisfaction scores for one agency can be compared to those of other agencies. In addition, many firms can perform more sophisticated statistical analyses of the data to help the agency set priorities for improvement, and can complete extensive "drill-down" analyses (such as analyzing differences in scores by various patient characteristics such as age, gender, and health status).

Home-care agencies that use a systematic approach to satisfaction measurement are able to focus limited resources on areas in need of improvement. Health-care consumers are exerting more influence than ever before, and are shopping for their health care and scanning research reports about local providers which review costs and quality. Agencies must prepare themselves for this new age of consumerism. As home-care agencies adopt systematic programs for patient-satisfaction measurement, providers and patients alike will reap the benefits of quality-improvement initiatives.

A Final Caveat

This article argues strongly for home-care managers to conduct ongoing evaluations of patient satisfaction. Home-care agencies are cautioned, however, that surveys are not a panacea. Using a survey does not mean that improvements will occur. While it is true that, "If you aren't measuring it, you aren't managing it," it is also true that "measuring isn't managing."

It is not enough for the home-care agency to observe that its patients aren't as satisfied with the concern for comfort demonstrated by nurses as are patients of other agencies. This data must be used to support actual changes in processes. Once a tested, reliable survey is implemented and management has meaningful data from which to draw basic conclusions, the real work of quality improvement is just beginning.

References

1. R. Baldor, *Managed Care Made Simple* (MA: Blackwell Science, Inc., 1996).
2. National Association for Home Care, *Basic Statistics About Home Care 1996* (Washington, DC).
3. D. Pontin and C. Webb, "Assessing Patient Satisfaction, Part I: The Research Process," *Journal of Clinical Nursing* (1995): 4(6):383—89.
4. B. Westra, L. Cullen, D. Brody, P. Jump, L. Geanon, and E. Milad, "Development of the Home Care Client Satisfaction Instrument," *Public Health Nursing* (1995): 12(6):393—99.

5. J. McCusker, "Development of Scales to Measure Satisfaction and Preferences Regarding Long Term and Terminal Care," *Medical Care* (1984): 22:476—93.
6. N. Risser, "Development of an Instrument to Measure Patient Satisfaction with Nurses and Nursing Care in Primary Care Settings," *Nursing Research* (1975): 24(1):45—52.
7. J.E. Ware, M.K. Snyder, R. Wright, and A.R. Davies, "Defining and Measuring Patient Satisfaction with Medical Care," *Evaluation and Program Planning* (1983): 6:247—63.
8. I. Press and M.F. Hall, "Monitoring Home Health Satisfaction," *Home Health Business Report* (September 1994): 15.
9. J.E. Ware, "Data Collection Methods," *Medical Outcomes Trust Bulletin* (January 1995): 2(6):2.
10. P. Shaughnessy, K. Grisler, R. Schlenker, and A.G. Arnold, "Outcome-Based Quality Improvement in Home Care," *Caring* (1995): 2:44—49.
11. C. Allred, P. Arford, and Y. Michel, "Coordination as a Critical Element of Managed Care," *Journal of Nursing Administration* (1995): 25(12):21—28.

APPENDIX A
Issues in Analyzing Home-Care Patient Satisfaction Surveys

As systematic approaches to home-care satisfaction become more prevalent, executives may need to update their own perceptions about how the data is presented. One common error is attempting to use the data to show how "well we are doing," as opposed to noting, "we have places to improve." This is best illustrated by the following example.

Let's say that a survey asked the question, "Likelihood of your recommending this agency," and used the five-point response scale below.

	Very Poor	Very Poor	Fair	Good	Good
	1	2	3	4	5

Now, consider three home-care agencies, each having 100 patients respond to the survey questions. The following are percentages of responses in each category. (These have been simplified to make the point.)

Agency 1	0%	0%	0%	50%	50%
Agency 2	0%	0%	0%	100%	0%
Agency 3	0%	0%	0%	0%	100%

Many analysts would report that home-care agencies 1, 2, and 3 have identical scores. (Each one has the scores of 100% if the responses in the "good" and "very good" categories are combined). For some audiences, each of the communities reporting 100% satisfied might be appropriate. However, most observers would easily regard Agency 3 as having the best results, and Agency 2 as having the worst.

Recent research suggests the notion that the distinction between the top two levels of responses is real. For example, Jones and Sasser believe "most managers should be concerned rather than heartened if the majority of their customers fall into the satisfied category" as opposed to the completely satisfied category.[6]

Another approach to working with the data is to assign points to the responses.

	Very Poor	Very Poor	Fair	Good	Good
Response	1	2	3	4	5
Points	0	25	50	75	100

Using the point assignment and the same percentages reported above, the three average scores (in points) for the agencies would be as follows.

Agency 1:	87.5 points
Agency 2:	75.0 points
Agency 3:	100.0 points

The distinctions between the level of satisfaction at the agencies are now more clear and match most observers' initial assessments. Press, Ganey Associates has adopted this approach to analyzing all its clients' surveys. Comparisons to the national databases are based upon the points scored by the agency.

About the Authors

Nancy Yezzi Moran, MS, RN, joined Press, Ganey Associates, Inc. in April 1995 as a Consultant for the firm's home health products. Nancy holds a BS in nursing and an MS in community health nursing. She is a graduate of Russell Sage College in Troy, NY. She has held professional positions in home health care for more than ten years. In previous positions Nancy has been the director of a hospital-based home health program, where she was responsible for budgetary and operational activities. Nancy has also worked for a free-standing non-profit home care agency, holding positions of supervising public health nurse and director of nursing. Nancy received board certification in enterostomal therapy; she was instrumental in implementing an enterostomal therapy nursing outpatient clinic. Other professional experience includes being responsible for all quality assurance activity, including JCAHO and regulatory compliance, of an outpatient facility. She is a member of Sigma Theta Tau and the American Nursing Association.

Mary P. Malone, MS, JD, CHE, is Vice President, Corporate Development at Press, Ganey Associates, Inc. Based in the firm's headquarters in South Bend, IN, she is responsible for the firm's strategic relationships, marketing and communications initiatives. Mary has consulted with hundreds of health care organizations, helping them to utilize patient satisfaction data in quality improvement initiatives. Mary received a MS in health systems management from Rush University and a JD from Notre Dame Law School. She holds a BS in biology and a BA in anthropology from the University of Notre Dame. She is a frequent author, speaker and commentator on issues related to patient satisfaction and is a diplomate in the American College of Healthcare Executives.

The authors gratefully acknowledge the assistance provided by Dennis O. Kaldenberg, PhD and Jennifer Cunnane in the preparation of this article.

Chapter 6

HOME-HEALTH QUALITY AND RESOURCE UTILIZATION IN A MANAGED-CARE ORGANIZATION

by Barbara Boyd, BSN, RN, Administrator, Home and Community Services, Group Health Cooperative of Puget Sound

Abstract
Home-health agencies owned by managed-care organizations confront the dilemma of providing quality patient care in an environment designed to control costs. While home health care is a strategy to assist managed-care organizations to achieve cost goals, providing good patient outcomes is equally important. Group Health Cooperative of Puget Sound is developing evidence-based systems to assure that the right amount of home health care is provided. Tools like Milliman and Robertson, Inc.'s home-care guidelines assist the home health-care department to move patients through the continuum of managed-care services. In addition, clinical outcomes, patient satisfaction, and cost/utilization ratios are optimized.

Introduction
Providing the right amount of home health-care services to individuals is both a challenge and a dilemma. The challenge comes from securing referrals in the highly competitive health-care environment. The dilemma is found in balancing the desires of the payer source with the needs of the individual patient. Currently, hospitals and some health-care organizations are using home-health services as a strategy to control costs. The use of this strategy is particularly true for managed-care organizations (MCOs) like Group Health Cooperative of Puget Sound (GHC). GHC owns and operates its own hospitals, skilled-nursing facility, home-health agency, and primary-care clinics. Even with this continuum of care options, GHC still faces the possibility of providing either too much or too little home health-care service. If access to home health care is limited, quality of care could be jeopardized and cost increased, especially if fewer home visits results in the increased use of high-cost acute medical care. Conversely, if home health-care services are allowed to go unmonitored, resources could be used far beyond the time when targeted patient outcomes are reached. The purpose of this article is to describe how GHC is developing

systems to assure that the right amount of home health care is being provided within its managed-care system. Specifically, the use of the Milliman & Robertson, Inc. (M&R) *Healthcare Management Guidelines* and their home-care guidelines at GHC is described.

GHC Home and Community Services
Headquartered in Seattle, Washington, GHC is the nation's largest consumer-governed health-care organization, serving a half-million people in the Pacific Northwest. While the majority of the GHC delivery system remains a staff model, GHC is increasing its network relationships. A founding characteristic of GHC was the integration of a financing mechanism with the delivery of health care. The result: GHC provides care within the discipline of a budget. However, GHC is not exempt from the competitive forces of the marketplace. GHC constantly debates how financial incentives affect patient outcomes and the health status of its enrollees.

Quality is a cornerstone at GHC, which received accreditation from the National Committee for Quality Assurance (NCQA) in 1996. GHC has a top-down commitment to quality improvement. Quality means everyone works all the time, every time, to meet or exceed the defined needs and expectations of patients and customers. This culture is shaped by the five beliefs listed in Appendix A.

Home and Community Services (HCS), a Medicare-certified and state-licensed home-health agency, exists within the GHC continuum of health-care services. HCS reflects the philosophy of the GHC managed-care environment. That is, patients move along a continuum of care, and the best quality and cost outcomes can be achieved when the right care is given in the right place, at the right time. Home-health outcomes are defined and measured as a part of GHC's care continuum.

GHC believes that reducing hospital days is the organization's greatest opportunity for savings. HCS contributes to the GHC savings in two distinct processes: First, as an alternative to length of hospital stay; and second, when home health care is used in place of a hospital admission. For example, one group of GHC primary-care clinics estimates that, in 1997, it will spend an additional $400,000 on home health care to save $1 million in hospital days. This decision will create a net savings to GHC of $600,000. Simultaneously, GHC and HCS believe that good patient outcomes will be sustained because care is provided safely and efficiently in the home setting.

Every GHC member chooses a personal physician who is part of a primary-care team. The team consists of one or more physicians, a physician's assistant or nurse practitioner, a registered nurse or licensed practical nurse, a medical assistant, and receptionist. The primary-care team acts as the entry point for care for each GHC member. Care is provided through the coordinated efforts of the primary-care team. Home-health services is an extension of the primary-care team's care plan.

The typical HCS patient is a female, over 70 years of age, who lives alone. The number of HCS patients served in 1995 and 1996 remained stable (Table 1). The number of home visits per patient increased slightly, as did the average length of stay in HCS.

Table 1
Patient Utilization of Home-health Services

	1995	1996
Number of Patients	7,683	7,770
Average Daily Census	866	1,143
Average Length of Stay (Days)	50	51
Average Visits/Admission	10	10.5

M&R Guidelines for Home Care

Milliman and Robertson (M&R) is one of the nation's leading consulting actuaries in health care. Their guidelines are experience-based descriptions of optimal recovery for a specific phase of patient care. In 1992, GHC began implementing M&R inpatient guidelines. The guidelines contain benchmark data that describe the optimal hospital length of stays by diagnosis. In 1995, HCS began consulting the M&R home-care guidelines.[1] The home-care guidelines describe the diagnosis, the number of home visits required for an optimally managed-care plan, and then the nursing interventions for each home visit.

Using the M&R home-care guidelines enables HCS to develop protocols and care pathways that maximize needed home-health interventions while minimizing the number of home visits. For instance, experience-based data show that when patients with congestive heart failure adhere to their medication regime, weigh themselves daily, and understand the signs and symptoms of an exacerbation of their disease process, they have fewer hospital admissions.[2] Using this data, M&R recommends that home-health providers focus on these interventions during home visits. Given these focused interventions, M&R guidelines suggest that the average congestive heart failure patient needs only up to three home-health visits.

M&R advocates that the primary-care clinic physician and/or the nursing case manager plan patient care in advance of care delivery. At GHC, primary-care clinic staff authorize patient care along the entire continuum. Consequently, HCS' personnel position themselves in the clinics. There they articulate the value of home visits for both resource expenditure and patient quality outcomes. Frequently, the HCS liaisons visit clinic physicians and attend weekly primary-care clinic meetings. The development of a personal relationship with physicians is crucial to the creation of trust and home-health nurses feeling like they belong to the clinic teams. It also sets the groundwork for the development of combined patient outcome evaluation processes.

Used together, M&R hospital and home-care guidelines pinpoint diagnosis groups where home health care can either decrease hospital length of stays or prevent admissions. For example, when GHC hospital length of stays were compared with M&R data, clear differences were present; GHC was using more hospital days than M&R recommended. In collaboration with primary-care team members, HCS used M&R home-care guidelines to identify interventions and home visits that could be substituted for hospital days. Currently, asthma, simple pneumonia, and congestive heart failure diagnoses are being evaluated. Because HCS is a major partner when hospital utilization strategies are developed, innovative HCS programs often evolve from these pathway, a home-health therapist makes one pre-surgical home visit. The following are achieved: a) evaluation of the home setting; b) determination of who will assist the patient at home following surgery; and c) demonstrations and practice with the patient/caregiver of toilet, bed, chair, and car transfers. The patient/caregiver are provided information on expected hospital length of stay and post-hospital regime. Following a post-operative hospital stay of two to three days, three to four home visits are made. Home health completes the physical assessments and obtains laboratory specimens. The physical therapist continues the strengthening and mobility physical therapy begun in the hospital. Care is then transitioned to independent follow-up by the physician and the physical therapist in the GHC primary-care clinic. For patients with co-morbidities that prevent them from getting to their primary-care clinic, post-surgical inpatient care extends beyond the three hospital days, and home health extends beyond the three to four home visits.

The M&R guidelines have limitations. Generally, M&R guidelines provide protocols to manage the uncomplicated patient, and they were built from experience with commercial populations. Commercial populations do not demonstrate the co-morbidity found in the Medicare population. Consequently, the M&R guidelines should not be implemented without reviewing an individual's specific condition and care needs. In the opinion of M&R, a patient with pneumonia requires three home-health visits; however, M&R does not consider the fact that the patient may have a co-morbidity of diabetes mellitus or chronic obstructive lung disease. GHC experience is that M&R guidelines are adequate for approximately 80% of the non-Medicare population and 50%

of the Medicare population. However, even if a care pathway is only adequate 50% of the time, it still builds the basis from which care can be delivered for the other 50% of the population.

HCS Quality Program
At GHC and HCS, quality is described in three ways: Quality of Care, Quality of Service, and Quality of Cost. Quality of Care describes health-improvement strategies, outcomes following an acute episode, or the rehabilitation process to reach an optimal functional status. Quality of Service describes patient satisfaction with the people who provided their care. Finally, Quality of Cost describes resource expenditures to obtain the quality of care and service.

HCS measures quality using two categories of quality indicators. The first category is universal, being used by all of GHC. For example, GHC measures Quality of Service by tracking the percent of members who rate care as "excellent for overall quality." For the overall quality indicator, 42% of the patients/families leave HCS give an excellent rating in overall quality. The HCS data for the indicator are included when GHC reports the data for the organization as a whole.

Second, HCS uses indicators that are specific to HCS programs. For example, in evaluating the Quality of Care and Quality of Cost for the total hip replacement care pathway, HCS does a program-specific analysis. A 10% random sample of charts is selected and audited. Variance from the care pathway and adherence to outlined pathway interventions are assessed. In addition, the cost for the HCS portion of the care is calculated. After the data are analyzed, a plan for improving either quality or cost is developed and implemented. Table 2 shows the total hip-care pathway indicators that were evaluated in 1995. HCS used the results to initiate quality-improvement activities during 1996.

Table 2
Total Hip-Care Pathway Indicators and Results for 1995

Indicator Results	Standard	Sample	Size
% Receiving Pre-op Home Visit	PT: 1 home visit	29	64%
% Receiving Post-op RN Home Visit	RN: 0—3 home visits	49	71%
Hydration Assessment	90% compliance threshold	37	75%
Vital Signs Assessment; Include Postural BP	90% compliance threshold	16	27%

Quality and Resource Utilization at HCS

In 1993, HCS combined quality and resource utilization through it definitions of Quality of Care, Service, and Cost. The combined goals are to achieve optimal clinical outcomes, to remain financially sound, and to obtain high scores in patient satisfaction with care and service. While M&R guidelines help HCS focus interventions and number of home visits, they do not provide criteria to measure whether optimal patient outcomes were achieved, nor do they measure the cost for each episode of care. Rather, M&R guidelines describe the number of visits and the interventions to be performed at the home visits. The interventions must be converted into specific patient outcomes in order to be used as quality indicators.

GHC manages care across a continuum of services in a manner which strives to obtain high scores in the three quality areas. Care plans must be constructed to maximize the efficiency of all care settings within the GHC continuum. M&R home-care guidelines inform HCS of the visits and the interventions, and, as a result, inform GHC as a whole. While quality is measured separately by care setting (e.g., hospital or home health), the measurements must be added together to create a comprehensive GHC picture of the three areas of quality. If M&R home-care guidelines are used to determine HCS's segment of care within the GHC care continuum, then HCS and GHC have the beginnings of an evaluation tool to measure patient outcomes along the whole continuum.

To illustrate, HCS developed a congestive heart failure care pathway based on experience and the M&R home-care guidelines. HCS determined that three to six home visits were needed for patients admitted with congestive heart failure. The care pathway described the interventions needed at each home visit and the patient outcomes and self-care behaviors. Using this care pathway, HCS plans to complete chart audits to measure compliance with both the number of home visits and patient interventions/outcomes. If patients consistently require more or fewer home visits to demonstrate the outcomes, the pathway will be altered to reflect the new, appropriate number of home visits. The audit will address both clinical outcomes and resource utilization. In the analysis, alternatives to home health can be evaluated. As needed, care can be shifted to either a lower level (e.g., the primary-care clinic) or a higher level (e.g., skilled-nursing facility). Quality, cost, and utilization data will assist the primary-care team to determine the amount of care and the best place for care.

To date, HCS has not performed these analyses. However, there are six care pathways which are ready for retrospective chart reviews. At the conclusion of these critiques, HCS plans to compare the number of home visits per admission versus the projected home visits prescribed by the care pathway. Information will also be available on some patient outcomes as well as HCS cost per episode of care.

By the end of 1997, HCS plans to move from a retrospective to a concurrent chart-review process. The new focus will allow HCS to evaluate, in real time, the effectiveness of the care pathways. For individuals on the care pathways, weekly records will be kept of the actual number of home visits, compared to the number of home visits the care pathway stipulates. The visiting nurse and his/her supervisor will use the visit data to trigger two possible care options.

First, the nurse consults the physician for the authorization of additional visits or for consideration of a higher care level for the patient. For example, the visiting nurse completes five days of twice-daily home visits to perform dressing changes. The care pathway indicates that, after the fourteenth day, the nurse must obtain consultation from a wound-care specialist. If the supervisor and the nurse were alerted to the situation, appropriate questions could be asked before a crisis on day fourteen. A conversation with the patient's physician might determine that admission to a skilled-nursing facility would be a more cost effective solution while achieving a better and more timely clinical outcome.

Second, the supervisor and nurse could have a discussion about why interventions were not performed or why the visit count is off schedule. The discussion gives an early alert to the supervisor, who can then assist the visiting nurse in either organization of the home visit or in performance improvement. Returning to the above situation, the visiting nurse may not be actively teaching a caregiver the wound care procedure, or his/her wound assessment skills may be sub-standard. The value of planned care with a concurrent audit process keeps the creative tension between cost and quality active and evolving in a timely way.

HCS is continually asked to scrutinize the number of home visits per patient that it is making. Using M&R as a template, then evaluating our own experience with visit numbers, clinical outcomes, and cost, HCS can assist the physicians to make data-driven decisions concerning the use of home health. HCS needs to be aggressive about not only the interventions required at each visit, but also the number of visits needed to assure that interventions are creating the desired outcomes. We are the experts in this arena, but intuition and anecdotal data are not adequate in this competitive health-care marketplace. Measurable care pathway outcomes are needed to equip HCS with the data to effect change of attitude as well as resource allocation.

Conclusion

GHC believes that cost and quality must exist in creative tension. Over the past several years, GHC has developed a growing body of work that demonstrates that the best quality health care also produces the best cost performance. GHC continues to move away from the traditional utilization-management programs toward strong care coordination and care planning. The M&R guidelines have been one tool used in this methodology. Built into these processes are strategies to achieve utilization targets as well as quality outcomes. The development of the systems and accountabilities is still work in progress.

HCS is assisting GHC to understand the relationship of the number of home visits and the interventions associated with the visits to the incidence of hospital readmissions or visits to the emergency department for a given diagnostic group. Together, a method to group care into diagnostic clusters is being developed. Using this technique, cost and utilization for the top 100 to 200 diagnostic categories can be analyzed across the continuum of care(e.g., inpatient, primary and specialty care, home health, and long-term care). Variations will be charted by primary-care clinics. In addition, for these same clinics, patient satisfaction and clinical outcomes will be monitored.

The task is not easy. GHC physicians, case managers, and HCS all agree that there is much more work to be done. The following questions must still be answered: a) Is HCS always the best alternative to a hospital stay? Would a skilled-nursing facility or sub-acute be more appropriate and less costly in the long run?; b) How is the number of home visits per HCS admission determined? Is M&R the only tool that should be used?; c) What are the best measures for patient outcome? Medical stability or functional?; d) How does HCS assist in building the extended care pathways to build a physician-driven comprehensive algorithm of care?; and e) What are the appropriate internal financing mechanisms that will maximize the movement of care across the continuum? Cost per visit or cost per case?

Given the rapid expansion of MCOs and the exponential growth of expenditures in home health, there is a critical need to examine the processes and outcomes of home-health services, to identify and test ideas for improvement, and to provide analysis and recommendations for change. We are all pioneers in this endeavor. HCS is being called upon not only to rethink its role in GHC's continuum of care, but also to re-examine the norms and behaviors which it must embrace. As a team member within a system of health care, home health must hold itself accountable for its part in obtaining cost effectiveness as well as the highest achievable patient outcomes.

References

Doyle, R.L., M.H. Pinney, and F.W. Spong. *Milliman & Robertson, Inc.yHealthcare Management Guidelines,* vol. 1, *Inpatient and Surgical Care.* (Milliman & Robertson: Author, 1994).

Doyle, R.L., M.H. Pinney, and F.W. Spong. *Milliman & Robertson, Inc. Healthcare Management Guidelines,* vol. 4, *Home Care and Case Management.* (Milliman & Robertson: Author, 1994).

APPENDIX A

Group Health Cooperative's Beliefs

I.	Patients' and customers' needs come first.
II.	Empowered teams and individuals meet customer/patient needs.
III.	People want to do their best and satisfy customers/patients.
IV.	Most problems are due to processes and systems, rather than people.
V.	Continuous improvement requires information, effort, support and time.

About the Author

Barbara Boyd received a B.S. in nursing from Pacific Lutheran University and has twenty-six years experience in the public health and home health areas. She has worked in a variety of program areas, including adult, maternal/child health, and hospice. Ms. Boyd was a Clinical Field Instructor in Public Health Nursing for California State University and has been with Group Health Cooperative of Puget Sound since 1988. She currently has administrative responsibility for Home Health, Hospice, Community Parent Child Services, AIDS Care Coordination, Home and Community Volunteer Services, and Referral Services. She is also in the second year of a Masters of Nursing program (MSN) at Seattle Pacific University.

Chapter 7

INITIATIVES AIM TO INTEGRATE PERFORMANCE MEASURES INTO THE JOINT COMMISSION'S ACCREDITATION PROCESS

by Maryanne Popovich, RN, MPH, Director, Joint Commission's Home Care Accreditation Services

The Joint Commission is continuing its efforts to implement changes that will modernize and improve the accreditation process for home-care and hospice organizations. Over the next few years, there are plans to formally introduce the use of performance measures and resulting data into the accreditation process. At the same time, the Joint Commission is encouraging home-care, hospice, and other health-care organizations to incorporate these measures into their own performance-improvement efforts.

Performance measures—quantitative measures used to evaluate and improve outcomes and the performance of functions and processes—are seen as being essential to the credibility of any modern evaluation activity for home-care and hospice organizations. Performance measures will supplement and guide the performance-based survey process by providing

- a more targeted basis for the regular Joint Commission accreditation survey;
- a basis for continuously monitoring actual performance; and
- a basis for guiding and stimulating continuous improvement in home-care and hospice organizations.

The Joint Commission envisions a process for including multiple performance-measurement systems in the future accreditation process, as well as a process for periodic solicitations of individual health-care performance measures from expert sources as well as provider organizations. The measures would support quality-improvement activities by measuring processes and/or outcomes of care, and could have wide applicability to all accreditation programs.

Catalogue of Performance Measures

The first major product of the Joint Commission's new approach to performance measurement is the *National Library of Healthcare Indicators*™ (*NLHI*™), a comprehensive indicator catalogue that includes performance measures judged by content experts to have face validity for application to various types of health-care organizations, including home-care and hospice organizations. This publication represents an effort to organize available and credible performance measures into a practical framework that can be easily used by health-care organizations, purchasers, and others. Ultimately, the Joint Commission hopes that *NLHI* will serve as a continuous source of promising indicators for performance-measurement systems.

In November, 1996, the Joint Commission released the first edition of *NLHI*, which includes performance measures for health-care networks and health plans. Future publications of *NLHI* will provide an expanded array of indicators applicable to the full range of health-care organizations, including home-care and hospice organizations. The Joint Commission will also routinely update and expand the measures already included in *NLHI*.

NLHI's performance measures are classified into three broad categories: priority clinical conditions arrayed against domains of performance; functional health status arrayed against clinical performance; and satisfaction from the perspectives of patients/enrollees, practitioners, and purchasers. The Joint Commission developed this classification system several years ago in collaboration with a group of major purchasers and providers.

Submitting Health-Care Indicators
The first edition of *NLHI* (*NLHI '96*) is based on the Joint Commission's first Request for Indicators (RFI), which focused on network and health-plan indicators. This yielded more than 900 suggested performance measures. A national panel of individuals having expertise in managed care considered those measures for inclusion in *NLHI* and selected 225 measures.

Measures from the second formal RFI for home care and hospice, ambulatory care, behavioral health care, and long-term care will be included in *NLHI '97*. As of fall, 1996, 16 organizations have submitted 185 home-care performance measures.

Periodically, the Joint Commission plans to issue RFIs to meet identified needs for indicators in specific areas of health care or for specific populations. In early 1997, a third formal RFI for hospital specialty services and pathology and clinical laboratories is planned. Subsequent RFIs are likely to address areas such as Medicare/Medicaid populations, critical care, geriatrics, and women's health.

Although the Joint Commission will continue to issue formal requests for performance measures, it welcomes the submission of indicators for potential inclusion in *NLHI* at any time. Examples of potential performance-measure topics for possible inclusion in *NLHI* have been developed for each of the Joint Commission's accreditation programs (home care and hospices, ambulatory care, behavioral health care, clinical laboratories, health-care networks, hospitals, and long-term care). (See Appendix A for comprehensive information on submitting home-care and hospice performance measures.)

However, topic areas for performance measures may transcend or cross accreditation programs and/or the three broad categories of clinical performance, health status, and satisfaction. For example, measures focused on Medicare or Medicaid populations could be applicable to any or all of the accreditation programs and/or broad categories.

Any entity or individual having interest and relevant expertise in measuring performance in health care may submit measures. Sources can include academic institutions, consumers, database developers, government or government-funded projects, health professionals, health-service researchers, insurers, performance-measurement systems, professional associations, provider organizations, and purchasers. Although RFIs are seen as a major source for potential inclusion in *NLHI*, measures from other sources such as established measurement systems will be included.

In selecting the indicators for *NLHI*, content experts judge the submitted indicators for face validity by asking questions such as, Does this performance measure address an important aspect of health care? and, How useful would this performance measure be in identifying opportunities to improve care?

Each indicator in *NLHI* has its own profile that defines the measure; describes its focus and rationale; details its characteristics, including risk adjustment and stratification, if any; portrays its applicability to various health-care delivery settings; and delineates the degree to which the indicator has been formally tested. Also included is information for contacting the organization or person who submitted the published performance measure.

Forms for submitting performance measures for consideration in *NLHI* are available by calling or writing the Joint Commission or on the Joint Commission's World Wide Web site. (See Appendix B for contact information.)

Evaluating Measurement Systems

The development of *NLHI* also is in line with the Joint Commission's goal of including multiple performance-measurement systems in the future accreditation process. In the next few years, the Joint Commission will require organizations—including home-care and hospice organizations—seeking accreditation to participate in an approved measurement system. However, organizations would be able to select from a group of approved systems to find the system or systems that best meet their needs.

The Joint Commission defines a performance-measurement system as an interrelated set of process measures, outcomes measures, or both that facilitates internal comparisons over time and external comparisons of an organization's performance. In 1995, the Joint Commission invited organizations to submit performance-measurement systems for evaluation for potential use in the future accreditation process. It then formed the Council on Performance Measurement, comprised of nationally known experts in performance measurement, who set out to recommend appropriate systems to the Joint Commission's Board of Commissioners.

Sixty-nine measurement systems formally requested consideration. Some of those submitted systems had a home-care focus. The council determined which systems had satisfied the initial criteria for participation in the accreditation process, and recommended those to the Board of Commissioners. The board considered approval of those systems at its January 1997 meeting.

At press time, the board was expected to select the systems to include in the future accreditation process. Once the board approves the systems, the Joint Commission is expected to release the approved list and begin a gradual process of implementation for health-care organizations seeking accreditation. Organizations would choose an approved measurement system and at least two specific performance measures from that system, and inform the Joint Commission of their selection.

An important underlying objective of this initiative would be to preserve the element of choice for accredited organizations. Specifically, the future requirements would permit organizations to select from a group of approved performance-measurement systems and find the system that would be best suited to their needs, and to select measures from that system that would be best matched to their patient population.

At press time, the planned implementation schedule called for hospitals and long-term care organizations to notify the Joint Commission of the systems they would be using by Dec. 31, 1997. In addition, to permit organizations ample time for planning and implementation, no data submissions for these types of organizations would be required until the first quarter of 1999.

The planned implementation schedule then called for home-care and hospice organizations, ambulatory-care facilities, behavioral health-care programs, laboratories, and health-care networks to chose an approved measurement system by Dec. 31, 1998, and begin to submit data sometime in late 1999 or early in the year 2000.

Planned time lines would be subject to adjustment based on assessments of field readiness. To ensure a smooth transition, the Joint Commission would provide health-care organizations with as much support and guidance as possible through this process.

The Joint Commission plans to make the review and approval of measurement systems an ongoing process. Additional performance-measurement systems would be approved over time, and approved systems would be monitored to ensure that they adhere to the established criteria as these continue to evolve in the future.

APPENDIX A
Request for Home-Care Performance Measures

The Joint Commission is seeking performance measures that cover the full spectrum of home care. Measures applicable to the following topic areas are being requested.

1. home care services
2. clinical conditions
3. home care patient-care processes
4. health/functional status
5. satisfaction
6. administrative/organizational functions

These topic areas will be refined and expanded as the unique measurement needs of home care are identified. Examples below are meant to be illustrative, not exhaustive.

1. Home care services *may* include
    - Nursing services
      — Private duty nursing
    - Home uterine monitoring
    - Personal care/support services
    - Pharmacy services
    - Infusion services
    - Laboratory services
    - Respiratory-care services
    - Home medical equipment services
      — Equipment delivery/service vehicles
    - Hospice services
    - Rehabilitation/therapy services
      — Rehabilitation technology services
    - Social-work services
    - Dietetic/nutritional services
    - Etc.

2. Measures of clinical conditions *may* include
    - Dementia care
    - Terminal care

- Chronic care
- Etc.

3. Measures of home care processes *may* include
    - Infection prevention and control
    - Medication and other therapeutic management
    - Patient/family/caregiver education
      — Preventive care
    - Etc.

4. Measures of health functional status *may* include
    - Cognition
    - Continence
    - Communication
    - Mobility
    - Self-care levels
    - Etc.

5. Measures of satisfaction *may* include
    - Patient/family/caregiver satisfaction
    - Payer satisfaction
    - Timeliness of visits
    - Scope and quality of services
    - Perceptions of respect
    - Etc.

6. Measures of administrative/organizational functions *may* include
    - Human-resource management
    - Information management
    - Staffing
    - Staff productivity
    - Costs per visit
    - Length of service
    - Fiscal viability
    - Unplanned inpatient admissions
    - Continuity of care.
    - Etc.

APPENDIX B
Contacts for Submitting Health-Care Performance Measures to the

National Library of Healthcare Indicators™
Department of Research and Evaluation
Request for Indicators Project
The Joint Commission on Accreditation of Healthcare Organizations
One Renaissance Boulevard
Oakbrook Terrace, IL 60181

Telephone: (630) 792-5971
Fax: (630) 792-5005
E-Mail: sprenger@jcaho.org

Joint commission World Wide Web site: http://www.jcaho.org
To access the submission forms follow these directions:
1. Click on the icon labeled "Enter The JCAHO Website"
2. Click on the icon labeled "Performance Measurement"
3. Click on the icon labeled "RFI"

About the Author

Maryanne Popovich, MPH, RN, is the Director of Home Care Accreditation Services at the Joint Commission of Accreditation of Healthcare Organizations. In this role, she is responsible for the operations of the Home Care Accreditation Program, including more than 4,000 accredited organizations and 166 surveyors. Before becoming the director of the Department of Home Care Accreditation Services, Ms Popovich served as an associate director in that department. She also has been a consultant surveyor for the Joint Commission. During her more than 20-year nursing career, Ms Popovich has held several clinical and managerial roles in a variety of home care and public health settings. Most recently, prior to joining the Joint Commission, Ms Popovich served as the chief executive officer for the Visiting Nurses Association of Crawford County in Meadville, Pennsylvania. In addition to her managerial roles, Ms Popovich has conducted numerous workshops and conferences regarding Quality Assurance and Performance Improvement in Home Care and Home Care Standards. Also, she has served as adjunct faculty at Theil College in Greenville, Pennsylvania and at the University of North Carolina, Chapel Hill. Ms Popovich earned her bachelor's degree in Nursing from Carlow College, Pittsburgh, Pennsylvania. In addition, she received her master's degree in Public Health from the University of North Carolina, Chapel Hill.

Chapter 8

THE CHAP BENCHMARKING PROGRAM: A SYSTEMATIC MEASUREMENT OF OUTCOMES TO ENHANCE RESOURCE UTILIZATION

by Theresa S. Ayer, MS, RN, CNAA, President and COO and Bernard Rose, Business Manager, Community Health Accreditation Program, Inc.

Introduction and Background
The Community Health Accreditation Program, Inc. (CHAP) is the oldest organization accrediting community and home-care agencies. It began providing this service in 1965, as part of the National League for Nursing (NLN), but in 1987 was separately incorporated.

CHAP is structured to demonstrate its commitment to quality and its belief that true quality can only be achieved by focusing on the needs of the consumer. CHAP is the only accrediting body in the nation that relies on standards of excellence to assess *all* areas of an organization, that is, client satisfaction, risk management, fiscal viability, and overall strength of management. Most importantly, CHAP is the only accrediting body in the nation that has offered full public access to accreditation findings, since its inception.

CHAP was the first national accrediting body to receive "deemed status" from the Health Care Financing Administration. In approving CHAP for "deemed status" in 1992, the federal government certified that CHAP's *Standards of Excellence for Home Care Organizations* met or exceeded the federal government's own standards for Medicare certification. As a result, CHAP-accredited organizations that receive deemed status are not subject to routine inspection by state survey agencies. CHAP-accredited organizations are "deemed" to meet Medicare Conditions of Participation because of their CHAP seal of approval.

The Ultimate Customer: The Consumer as an Active Player in Care
Customer needs and desires for their own care have become an undeniably important part of defining quality of care—a quality that had previously been defined only by provider and payer values and goals. Health-care reform is happening even without legislative action. The legislative efforts have, however, brought a new awareness to consumers. The attention has repositioned patients and encouraged them to become "empowered" consumers, often

directing their own care. In this climate, no home-health agency can survive and succeed without incorporating the needs and values of this ultimate customer, and what this patient needs and wants to achieve through their care.

Compared to other components in the continuum of health care, home care has a unique problem with respect to client satisfaction: Caring for a consumer at home does not just mean maintaining that person's health and functional ability in an objectively defined way, it also means maintaining his or her personal lifestyle to a far greater extent than is possible in any residential long-term care setting. Home care is the one health-care setting in which the provider comes into the patient's or client's domain rather than vice versa.

Quality of *life* can really be a dimension separate from quality of *care*, yet fundamental to a client's well-being and to the whole philosophy of in-home care. Quality of life is idiosyncratic to the client and, at first glance, conflicts with the notion of uniformity of standards and procedures. Yet, to achieve quality-of-life objectives means finding criteria not unique to each client. It is here that a system of defined, consumer-based outcome measures can directly assure this goal. Benchmarks developed through research with consumers can sufficiently delineate areas important to many individuals so as to make this possible.

Theorists have generally recognized three basic, traditional categories of quality-of-care standards in health care: structural, process, and outcome measures. Outcome measures are concerned with the end result of care—whether there is any measurable change (or stabilization) in the health or social status of the patient as a result of services rendered. Outcome measures are obviously easier to develop where there are discrete, changeable physical conditions being examined, as is common in hospitals or other acute-care settings. Outcome measurements for home-health clients with acute or chronic conditions are impacted by mental, physical, and/or functional limitations, and are harder to develop.

Consumers play the most important role in achieving positive outcomes. Consumers are the only constant in an ever evolving and rapidly changing health-care system. Governmental policy can change, provider response to regulation and service configuration may change, the range of services offered by HMOs/MCOs can change, insurers and payers may change, accreditation organizations responding to all of the above will change, but consumer needs for improved outcomes and well-being will never change. Therefore, the responsibility to incorporate consumer input into the process of improving health outcomes carries intense and sometimes burdensome accountability. How do those entrusted to serve and protect the well-being of a nation respond?

The answer to this question is to produce positive outcomes, as determined by the ultimate customer, who, in effect, is the home-health consumer. How many times has the health-care professional determined what is right for the consumer, only to be frustrated with the outcome because the consumer has not participated in the delivery of their care? The lack of consideration for a consumer's environment, cultural or social beliefs, ethical or moral values, religious or educational background, mental or psychological state, race, creed, color, and/or sexual preference all impact on positive outcomes. All of these factors will contribute to positive or negative health-care outcomes, although some weigh more heavily than others. How does the health-care professional integrate these interests into the plan of care?

Outcomes must therefore be viewed holistically. How does an organization balance the competing interest and the potential conflict of consumer participation in their plan of care? How are the professional's expertise and the consumer's expectations integrated into the plan of care to produce quality outcomes? How are outcomes or performance measured? What performance measures should be incorporated into an organization's quality-improvement process? How are quality performance measures linked to outcomes in the allocation of resources? How should quality performance measures relate to national accreditation standards and improved outcomes?

Quality: An Ever-Evolving Vision
Quality is no different than the old adage, "beauty is in the eye of the beholder." Quality is in the eye of the beholder—anyone can judge quality according to their definition. The beholder, to be totally objective, needs nationally recognized standards to gauge quality of performance.

Unless quantified, quality is subjective. Quality is open to debate by consumer, payer, provider, and any oversight body. Quality, therefore, is ever evolving—it is not static, but rather dynamic. Quality is not rigid but flexible—able to integrate a holistic view by empowering *all involved*. Quality, as a result, is not precisely definable, but rather flexible enough to change with the winds of time.

Hence, quality is a vision that guides a process and forms the foundation for those who attempt to define "quality." Therefore:

- Quality is determined by the consumer, who is, in effect, the ultimate customer.
- Quality is the responsibility of management, but is everyone's job. All employees own quality; it is an internal value that can be taken wherever one goes.

- Quality is produced by an empowered employee. An empowered worker has the authority to do what needs to be done to get the job done at that time. Coupled with this authority is the accountability of all employees.
- Quality is a concurrent process. Rather than being reactive, it is proactive, and an ongoing strategy.
- Quality is measured holistically and is larger than the sum of its parts.

    a) The quality of a consumer's care has to be viewed in relationship to their beliefs and values, their family, and their environment. The parts (e.g., wound healing, range of blood sugars, etc.) have significance only within the context of this greater whole.

    b) Quality is the interaction between the user and the producer of a service. Thus, producing quality home care must take into consideration both the consumer and an organization's staff members. Therefore, quality is measured by looking at *all outcomes* as a whole. No one outcome by itself signifies quality.

- Quality is a focus on the positive and the development of excellence in caregivers. People are the driving force in quality.
- If people do not provide quality care, it is usually because of a problem in the system in which they work.
- Quality is data-supported, not data-driven. Data provided are for learning rather than as evidence of "poor performers or performances".
- Quality means maximizing human, physical, and financial resources so that services are enhanced.

This unique approach to health-care delivery is different from our traditional thinking about outcomes, and the accountability shared by consumers and providers. For example, insurers base reimbursement on quantitative values, such as whether the organization has justified reimbursable services according to their criteria. There is an apparent absence of consumers' participation in defining what is acceptable care or quality. Empowering and informing consumers of their responsibilities for participating in choices about their care is an essential aspect of effective delivery of quality care.

Defining Quality: Elusive as the Limits of the Universe
While the meaning of quality is universal, the definition of quality is open to many interpretations. Whether those interpretations are clearly understood or quantified is open to further explanation. The *Benchmarks for Excellence in Home Care* program is not the definitive statement on quality, but it attempts to refocus the discussion. By incorporating the consumer and a holistic view of what quality outcomes should produce, this program establishes new param-

eters for continued positive dialogue that should lead to improved outcomes—both for the consumer and for the organization that engages the program and process.

Defining Quality Requires Empirical Research
Defining quality in home health care is as elusive as understanding the mysteries of the universe. Peter Shaughnessy, PhD, and CHAP, however, have this task well begun. Dr. Shaughnessy is a professor at the University of Colorado Health Sciences Center in Denver and Director of the Center for Health Services Research. While both have taken a different approach, the conclusions regarding the empirical data will be similar.

Dr. Shaughnessy has focused on the clinical performance measures that impact upon outcomes, while CHAP has taken a more holistic view of outcomes. Dr. Shaughnessy's clinical measures are both comprehensive and well defined, and are becoming the clinical standard for the home health-care industry. CHAP, while interested in the factors that impact upon clinical outcomes, believes that multiple factors drive outcomes—not just clinical factors.

CHAP's holistic view led it to attempt to quantify these multiple factors. CHAP initiated a process with the support and underwriting of funds from the W.K. Kellogg Foundation and the National League for Nursing (NLN). CHAP received a $1.2 million grant from the W.K. Kellogg Foundation in 1989 to develop consumer-oriented outcome measures for the home-care industry. The NLN, CHAP's parent organization, also invested considerable resources in supporting this innovative project. The culmination of seven years of research resulted in the development of a state-of-the-art self-evaluation computer-software package, *Benchmarks in Excellence in Home Care*. This data-management system assists organizations in determining their level of performance in specific areas. The software provides organizations with a detailed map of service quality that focuses on outcomes and includes resource utilization in its measures of quality.

All organizations and entities agree that quality indicators are essential to defining quality outcomes. The question then becomes: How do we know we have quality indicators?

Defining Quality Indicators
Our traditional thinking in health care regarding the definition of quality indicators has focused on the organization or the array of services it provides. Clearly, there has been an absence of both consumers and their expectations. Organizations have been directed by regulatory pressures to define quality based on monitoring high-volume activities, low-volume activities, or high-

risk activities. Because of the fluidity of these regulatory pressures, seldom have organizations stopped to question the rationale for such determinations.

Regulatory pressures are politically motivated and there is a dearth of consumer contribution. Today, however, the consumer has become an active participant in the delivery of care, and quality indicators must therefore incorporate consumer perceptions and concerns. Their attitudes, beliefs, and opinions are important ingredients that impact upon quality outcomes. The definition of what constitutes quality outcomes includes consumer empowerment and satisfaction. The degree of motivation, for example, can assist or hinder a patient's recovery, thereby impacting on outcomes, consumption of resources, and an individual's health status. Quality is best evaluated by quantitative parameters that measure improvements through consumer-focused outcomes.

Holistic Definition of Quality
CHAP's initial research in the "In Search of Excellence in Home Care" project defined three aspects of quality: the consumer, the staff or caregivers, and the organization. Outcomes can only be evaluated over time, with clearly articulated goals that have been established between the consumer and caregiver. It is the responsibility of the caregiver to provide consumers with the knowledge and information necessary to make informed decisions about their care. Finally, the relationship between the financial strength and viability of an organization impacts on the quality of service provided.

These were the three aspects of quality that resulted in the first three benchmarks for home health care. Subsequent industry input indicated that these aspects should be broadened to include a more holistic view of an organization, and so outcome measures were developed for financial operations and risk management.

The Evaluation of Quality Performance Through Outcome Measurement
One of the most daunting tasks faced by health-care providers today is how to find meaningful indicators that will yield information to measure and improve outcomes to enhance quality. CHAP's commitment to quality home care through standards with a strong consumer focus led to its development of an outcomes measurement tool for home care. The research that began the process included, as an integral part, the identification of what was important to consumers. The Kellogg grant obtained by CHAP allowed it to conduct groundbreaking research that resulted in a system of benchmarks, or outcome measures, for home care.

Benchmark ratings are a powerful tool for assessing the strengths and weaknesses of an organization, and for seeing where an organization stands in relation to the industry as a whole. These ratings can be used to drive internal quality improvement, and to secure both industry and consumer recognition. Benchmark ratings highlight problem areas, so that quality-improvement efforts, including resource allocation, can be directed where they are most needed. By providing a focused vision of what home care should provide, a benchmarking program gets everyone aiming at the same mark.

Benchmarking, or outcomes measurement, can assist in resource utilization by helping an organization validate its quality-improvement efforts. Benchmarking activities can provide a quantifiable profile of an organization's services to use for identifying areas where reallocation of resources can make the most difference. Benchmarking can also assist in increasing consumer satisfaction by focusing resources on areas that are most important to an organization's clients.

Benchmarks and Outcome Measures in Home Care
The five benchmarks developed by CHAP, named "Pulse Points," became the software program *Benchmarks for Excellence in Home Care*. The original research included data from 2,006 consumers, 1,909 home-care staff, and 138 managers, and formed the basis for a national database. Consumers, home-health caregivers, and organizational staff provided invaluable information and guidance in the development of tools that are sensitive to the home health-care industry. The three primary goals of the Kellogg research project were as follows.

- To design a methodologically valid and reliable instrument with which to assess consumer attitudes regarding the quality of health services received in the home.
- To develop a system for collecting and reporting relevant information, to allow for meaningful comparisons over time between agencies as well as within agencies.
- To develop empirically sound outcome measures of quality for all elderly patients (over 65) in home health care.

CHAP's *Benchmarks for Excellence in Home Care* program provides home-care organizations with precise data-collection instruments, questionnaires, and tools to assist in the collection of data that provides a basis for internal quality-improvement initiatives. The collected data is returned to CHAP and is linked to an analysis program that provides aggregate scores for three of the five benchmarks of quality. These benchmarks, or Pulse Points, circumscribe a basic category for defining and measuring quality in home care.

Originally, the Kellogg Research project, "In Search of Excellence in Home Care," defined three Pulse Points: Consumer Satisfaction, Clinical Services, and Organizational Management. These were expanded to five Pulse Points, with the addition of Financial Management and Risk Management, in 1995. This resulted in the broadly based, holistic map of an organization's operations produced by the current *Benchmarks for Excellence in Home Care* program. Each Pulse Point has multiple "Indicators"—types of information accessed by the questionnaires and data-collection instruments developed for that Pulse Point. These Indicators are further divided into "Probes" that define the parameters of a particular Indicator. There are 28 Indicators in all.

CHAP's research determined, through the input of providers and consumers, and industry analysis, that to fully assess an organization's quality performance, the organization needs to be viewed holistically. Taken in their totality, these Pulse Points, their Indicators, and the defining Probes represent a holistic view of organization operations and their accompanying outcomes. The five Pulse Points and their Indicators follow.

I. **Consumer Pulse Point**

Outcome: Recording consumer responses to identify their satisfaction with agency. Comparisons will show the effects of interventions as perceived by the client.

Indicators measured:
1. Consumer Empowerment
2. Relationship Between Consumers and Caregivers
3. Knowledge/Information Needed by the Consumer
4. Family Support
5. Consumer Expectations of the Provider

II. **Clinical Pulse Point**

Outcome: Measuring physiological parameters, such as vital signs, ability to do own ADLs, and other behavioral outcomes. Comparisons will show the effects of clinical interventions by measuring the health status on admission and any changes that have occurred at discharge.

Indicators measured:
6. Empirical Indicators of Consumer's Functional Ability
7. Physiological Indicators of Consumer's Functional Ability

III. **Organizational Pulse Point**

Outcome: Measuring staff and management responses to identify their commitment to quality, teamwork, and organizational coordination of care.

Indicators measured:
8. Team-Building
9. Commitment to Quality
10. Coordination of Care

IV. Financial Management Pulse Point

Outcome: Financial resources and systems support the service needs of the home-care organization and its consumers in a cost-effective manner, and ensure the financial viability of the organization.

Indicators measured:
11. Liquidity Ratios and Calculations
12. Profitability Ratios and Calculations
13. The Viability-Score Calculation (V-Score)
14. Efficiency Ratings
15. Productivity Ratios
16. Cost
17. Utilization

V. Risk Management Pulse Points

Outcome: The home-care organization has tracking and trending processes and systems in place in order to determine whether any of its current practices increase the exposure of the consumer and the organization to liability. When such threats are detected, the organization implements affirmative measures to minimize risk.

Indicators measured:
18. Infection Rate Monitoring
19. Injury Occurrence
20. Incident Reporting
21. Potential Malpractice
22. Nutritional Management
23. Intake Assessment
24. Claims Management and Recognition
25. Continuity of Equipment, Supplies, and Medications
26. Financial Management
27. Contract Execution and Review
28. Adverse Drug Reactions and Medication Incidents

These Pulse Points measure the many dimensions of quality in home care as they are found in CHAP's *Standards of Excellence for Home Care Organizations* and the HCFA Conditions of Participation. Throughout the *Benchmarks for Excellence in Home Care* program, these two sources provide the foundation for specific questionnaires, data-collection instruments, Indicators, and Probes. They also convey the philosophy of excellence that has long driven CHAP.

Benchmarking and Resource Utilization

How an organization manages its resources, whether service is delivered effectively and efficiently, is crucial to its success and long-term viability. Benchmarks are designed to improve systems and processes, and facilitate the identification of effective resource allocation. For example, the number of home visits made to a client with congestive heart failure can often be decreased through focus on consumer-empowerment activities. Often, the client is overwhelmed by the medical regime and does not "hear" what the nurse is teaching (Martens, et. al., 1997). While this is news to nurses in the field, the ability to quantify the most important factors to a particular population of clients can assist in the development of specific care plans.

Another perspective on the same situation is the ability to quantify needs, concerns, and areas of importance to the client. Once an organization has quantifiable data, it has a tool for demonstrating to managed-care organizations the long-term value of additional visits in the short term. A client who becomes compliant with a special diet and medications will save the managed-care organization money in the prevention of future hospitalizations. Home-care staff have known this for years, but it is only recently that techniques for outcomes management have become available. Using benchmarking as a tool for deciding how to allocate and reallocate resources will facilitate organizational goal attainment.

A comprehensive evaluation of adequate resources must include human, financial, and physical resources. To be most efficiently organized for today's extremely competitive market, a home-health agency must use every available tool to identify how best to allocate resources. Only in this way can an organization fulfill its stated mission. The corollary to this key quality-improvement principle implies that the management and governing authority provide the organization with the tools necessary to provide quality service. Thus, there must be an overall organizational commitment to the provision of quality resource allocation. Staff, in turn, must demonstrate a commitment to empowerment through team-building and the organizational coordination of care for overall consumer satisfaction.

Summary
CHAP clearly believes that any process that attempts to improve outcomes, and thereby resource utilization, must incorporate the consumer as the apex of its efforts. Consumer values, whether social, cultural, or any other, must be the driving force in improving outcomes. If community and home-health programs fail to incorporate and involve the consumer in the choices about their care, then whose interest is being served—the consumer's or the industry? CHAP has long weighed in on the side of the consumer to make community and home health care an important, essential, and viable option in the health-care debate.

Allocating resources to keep consumer service and profitability in equilibrium will insure every agency long-term success. Outcome measures only affect the quality of care if they are a part of quality programs. This is, perhaps, the most urgent reason for the incorporation of outcome measures into daily practice.

An organization's financial viability and growth are, to a large extent, dependent on how it allocates its resources. Using quantifiable parameters allows the organization to justify its decisions, with respect to resources, to governing bodies, physicians, and managed-care organizations.

References

CHAP. *In Search of Excellence in Home Care—Final Report to W.K. Kellogg Foundation.* (1994).

CHAP. *Benchmarks for Excellence in Home Care—Operator's Tutorial.* (1996).

Department of Health and Human Services, Health Care Financing Administration. "Medicare Program: Recognition of the Community Health Accreditation Program Standards for Home Care Organizations." *Federal Register* (May, 1992): 57(104):22,773–80.

Martens, K.H. and S.D. Mellor. "A Study of the Relationship Between Home Care Services and Hospital Readmission of Patients With Congestive Heart Failure." *Home Healthcare Nurse* (1997): 15(2):123–29.

National League for Nursing and Community Health Accreditation Program. (1997). *Standards of Excellence for Home Care Organizations.* New York: Author.

Shaughnessy, P.W., et. al. "Measuring and Assuring the Quality of Home Health Care." *Health Care Financing Review* (1994): 16(1):35–67.

About the Authors

Theresa S. Ayer, MS, RN, is the current President and Chief Operating Officer of the Community Health Accreditation Program, Ind. (CHAP), a subsidiary of the National League for Nursing. CHAP is an independent, consumer-driven not-for-profit corporation that has been assessing the quality of home and community health organizations since 1965. Prior to joining CHAP in April 1996 as Interim President, Ms Ayer was Vice President for Programs at the VNA of Northern Virginia, Inc., where she had worked for over eight years. She has worked in home and community health since 1980 with all types of organizations—home health, private duty and public health agencies that were proprietary, non-profit and governmental. Since 1990 Ms Ayer has also consulted as a CHAP site visitor. Ms Ayer earned her masters degree in health care administration from Central Michigan University, and her BSN from Wright State University in Dayton, Ohio. She is also certified in advanced nursing administration.

Bernard Rose is the Business Manager for the Community Health Accreditation Program, Inc. (CHAP). Prior to joining CHAP in 1995, Mr. Rose was the principal in Rose Consulting Group. Mr. Rose was the Executive Director at Kings County Hospital Center in Brooklyn, N.Y. and at Helen Hayes Hospital in West Haverstraw, N.Y. He has an extensive health care background in both hospital and community care settings. He has held appointments to the Governor's Task Force on Technology and the Disabled and the Health Commissioner's Task Force on Health Manpower and Labor Productivity. Mr. Rose holds a bachelor's degree from Manhattanville College in Purchase, N.Y. and has attended New York University's School of Public Administration.

Chapter 9

PROSPECTIVE PAYMENT: IMPACT ON RESOURCE UTILIZATION AND QUALITY

by Karen Beckman Pace, MSN, RN
Vice President, Research, and Regulatory Affairs
National Association for Home Care

Abstract

Prospective payment for Medicare home-health services is likely to be enacted in the near future. The Health Care Financing Administration (HCFA) and the home-care industry are committed to a per-episode prospective payment system (PPS) with payment based on an episode or period of care rather than a visit.

Moving to PPS represents a major change not only in the payment mechanism, but also in how agencies manage the care of home-health patients. Under a PPS, providers have more flexibility in care management, since reimbursement is not tied to visits. But home-care agencies are at financial risk if the costs of providing care exceed the set payment rates.

The movement toward PPS occurs in a time of increased accountability for quality. The changes brought about by PPS have the potential to be positive or negative, depending on the strategies taken by home-care providers. The ultimate goal is to provide quality care for the least cost. Outcome measures are an important tool for measuring the impact of changes in care practices as well as for helping identify the most efficient ways to provide care.

Success under PPS will require providers to integrate clinical and financial data. They will need to carefully examine the relationship between costs, utilization of services, care practices, and the outcomes of care to determine the appropriate strategies to undertake.

Prospective payment for Medicare home-health services is likely to be enacted in the near future. This represents not merely a change in payment mechanism, but a total culture change for most home-care organizations. The change in financial incentives may influence care practices and quality of care. However, these changes are not necessarily negative or positive; they have the potential to be either, depending upon the home-care organization's response to the incentives and basic commitment to providing quality services.

A prospective payment system (PPS) is a method of reimbursement whereby the payment rate is known in advance of delivering the service. A PPS can be based on a variety of units of payment, such as per-visit, per-episode, per-enrollee, or per-outcome. The home-care industry and the Health Care Financing Administration (HCFA) are committed to implementing a per-episode PPS. The advantages of per-episode PPS include curtailing increases in utilization; promoting cost containment; allowing flexibility in care management; eliminating retroactive cost disallowances that can occur with cost reimbursement; and rewarding agencies for being efficient.

With a per-episode PPS, home-care providers are reimbursed for an episode of care, rather than for each visit provided. The "episode" for a national payment system has not yet been defined. In the current HCFA demonstration testing a per-episode payment methodology, an "episode" is defined as 120 calendar days following admission[1]. A new episode is not recognized until there is a period of 45 days without covered home-health services. A new HCFA study to develop a case-mix system for home-health PPS is designed to explore various time periods for the episode.

Per-Episode PPS
Under per-episode reimbursement, patients are categorized according to a case-mix classification system so that reimbursement reflects the costs of providing service to a particular category of patients. "Case mix" refers to the characteristics of patients served that influence the cost of care, such as age, functional impairment, and severity of medical condition. An individual patient's care may be more or less costly than the set payment rate. However, the per-episode reimbursement rate should reflect the cost of providing care for a specific patient group closely enough to prevent the incentive to refuse care to certain types of patients.

Per-episode reimbursement presents opportunities and challenges to home-care providers. It offers more flexibility in managing patient care, since reimbursement is not tied only to making visits. In addition, with per-episode payments, visits are viewed as costs to be managed rather than revenues, as in fee-for-service reimbursement. Agencies will seek to find patterns of care and mix of services that are most efficient for providing home-health services. Some options that home-care providers can explore include telephone follow-up, tele-health applications, making visits prior to hospital discharge, and making longer but less frequent visits. With prospective payment, home-care providers will find themselves operating in much the same manner as case mangers or managed-care organizations, in that they will be trying to provide care at the lowest possible cost. However, the Medicare benefit and coverage guidelines will remain the same. Utilization of services will have to be managed within the

Medicare coverage guidelines. For example, patients who need personal-care services and do not have an able or willing caregiver are entitled to home health-aide services[2]. The aide services should be provided even if that care may result in costs above the set payment rate or limit.

If home-care services are provided for less than the set episode reimbursement rate, agencies may experience a profit. On the other hand, if costs are higher than the set payment rate, agencies may suffer a financial loss. It is critical for home-care providers to "manage" the care provided to patients so that, on average, they maintain the cost of care below the payment rate. Effective management will require an integration of clinical and financial processes, data, and staff.

The major obstacle to implementing a per-episode PPS is the lack of an effective case-mix system. The current case-mix adjustor used in the HCFA demonstration accounts for less than 10% of the variation in cost among Medicare home-health patients[3]. Without an adequate case-mix adjustor, agencies may reject caring for patients with costly care requirements. Recently, HCFA initiated a new, 30-month study to develop a case-mix classification for a home-health per-episode PPS. The case-mix study uses the Outcome and Assessment Information Set (OASIS), which HCFA plans to implement for measuring outcomes in home-health agencies, and some additional data items considered to be predictive of home-care service use[4].

Because of the current political and economic environment and the threat of major reforms in Medicare, the home-care industry is supporting PPS as an alternative to co-payments for Medicare home-health services or bundling home-care services with hospital DRG payments. The industry's Unified Proposal for PPS (see Appendix 1) begins with an interim system based on per-visit payments subject to aggregate limits, and culminates in per-episode PPS with an improved case-mix system.

An Interim PPS

The industry's interim system has two phases. In Phase I, payment is based on prospectively set per-visit payment rates for each discipline, subject to an agency's annual aggregate per-patient limit. Phase II also uses the set per-visit payment rate. There is an agency annual aggregate episode limit for days 1 through 120 in an episode, and an agency annual aggregate per-patient limit for visits after 120 days. In both Phases I and II, home-care agencies share in any savings achieved if payments are below the agency's aggregate limit. The agency's share of the savings is equal to 50% of the savings, up to a maximum of 10% of their reimbursement, with some limitations related to the per-patient limits.

The per-patient limit in Phase I and post-120-day per-patient limit in Phase II are based on an agency's historical case mix and costs per patient, blended with the census-region experience. An agency's historical cost-per-patient data is used because it reflects the mix of patients cared for by that agency. And, in general, an agency's case mix does not change radically over time. The blend with census-region data requires the most inefficient agencies to bring costs more in line with the region, and provides some flexibility and opportunity for reward for the most efficient agencies. The per-episode limits in Phase II use the HCFA per-episode demonstration case-mix adjustor and are based on the utilization experience by case-mix category in a metropolitan statistical area (MSA) or non-MSA.

Financial Incentives
In the interim system, the financial incentives are twofold: a) to decrease the unit cost per visit per discipline, and b) to decrease the overall case cost, or cost per patient served. If the agency's cost per visit is below the set payment rate, the difference is retained. For example, if an agency's cost for a skilled-nursing visit is $84 and the set payment rate is $85, the agency makes $1 on each nursing visit. If the agency's total payment is below the aggregate limit, it receives 50% of the savings up to a maximum of 10% of the reimbursement. For example, if the agency's aggregate limit is $1 million and their payment equaled $900,000, their share of the savings will be $50,000 (half of $100,000). In a per-episode system, the financial incentive is to keep aggregate costs below the aggregate episode payments to retain the difference between cost and payment. The episode cost is a function of the number of visits, cost per visit, and other types of services provided, such as through tele-home-care mechanisms. Consequently, agencies still must manage both the cost of providing services and service utilization.

Viewed in isolation, financial incentives could drive a decrease in the number of visits provided, which may ultimately impact quality. That is, an agency stands to make a profit by simply providing fewer services than those services used to determine the aggregate limit or per-episode payment rate. A PPS also creates incentives to lower the cost of providing services, such as personnel costs, supplies, travel, and documentation time.

Curbing utilization and costs are intended effects of a PPS from the payer's perspective. But reducing the number of visits and costs can lead to either greater efficiency or poorer quality, depending upon the strategies and extent of cost-cutting measures employed by the agency. The "right amount" of visits to produce desired outcomes for particular types of home-care patients is unknown at this time. Significant variation in utilization exists across the country. It is unwise to simply choose the average or the lowest number of visits without more information on differences in patients served and the result of the care received. Patients who receive the higher levels of care may be adversely affected by reducing care to the average or lowest amount. Only by studying the interaction of utilization, cost, patient characteristics, and outcomes of care, can the appropriate level of care be determined.

Most home-care providers will not respond to purely financial incentives. Home-care providers will continue to strive to provide quality services within the financial constraints of the reimbursement system. If the payment system is inadequate to reimburse agencies for the cost of providing covered services to Medicare beneficiaries, no amount of management will result in quality care. But if reimbursement is based upon reasonable expectations of the cost of providing services, then the goal is to find the level of service required to produce quality care for a cost that is at or below set payment limits or rates.

The home-care industry's PPS proposal recognizes the potential for abusive practices and includes provisions to identify and prevent negative incidents. Beneficiary due-process procedures will allow patients to challenge care and coverage determinations. Quality reviews are triggered for significant variations in utilization, as when an agency suddenly and dramatically decreases the average number of visits provided to the patients served.

Managing Utilization and Cost
Ultimately, success under PPS depends upon adequately managing costs and utilization of services to achieve appropriate patient outcomes. Success requires skill in accurately identifying costs, managing utilization, and measuring and interpreting outcomes to influence care practices resulting in quality care.

Typically, utilization data include visit information. At a minimum, utilization information requires numbers of visits by type of discipline, such as nursing, physical therapy, and aide. Home-care providers need to develop the capacity to analyze utilization data in a variety of ways, such as per admission, per patient per year, and per episode. Each of these presents specific data issues. Reporting utilization by admission requires precise and standard definitions of admission and discharge. Statistics reported per patient per year require the ability to identify "unduplicated" patients—that is, each individual served is counted only once in the calendar year, regardless of the number of admissions. Episode information requires a definition of when an episode begins and ends, for example after a 45-day period without Medicare-reimbursed home-health services. In addition, utilization data should be analyzed by diagnosis, payer source, and case-mix category. As agencies move away from visits as the basis of all care, they will need to look at other measures of utilization, such as the time spent with the patient in visits, coordination, and telecommunication.

In order to adequately manage costs and select appropriate strategies, the home-care organization needs accurate cost data. Costs need to be properly allocated to the various programs and services. For example, allocating a supervisor's salary across several programs would be based on the actual time and activity devoted to each program, rather than some percentage distribution based on visits or revenues for each area.

Managing Quality
The home-care industry will implement a PPS in an era not only of cost containment, but also of accountability for quality. Quality reflects the home-care agency providing the appropriate services, safely and competently, within the appropriate time frame, and achieving the desired patient outcomes, that can be influenced by the services provided[5]. Today, quality initiatives are focused on objective performance indicators with an emphasis on patient outcomes, and outcome measurement is critical to successfully implementing PPS.

The term "outcome" may be used to denote a variety of dimensions, including cost, utilization of services, goals of care, and actual patient condition. However, in the context of quality, a patient outcome represents a change in health status between two or more points in time. Health is considered broadly and encompasses both physical and psychosocial aspects of the patient. Sometimes utilization of health services such as emergency-room visits are used as a proxy for more difficult-to-measure clinical outcomes. Outcome measurement is an attempt to quantify the effect of rendered care.

Measuring outcomes helps identify the effects of cost-cutting strategies and decreased utilization of services on the patients served. Outcomes will be of interest to providers, consumers, payers, and policy makers. Outcomes are also a tool for providers to identify the most cost efficient methods of providing care under a PPS—that is, how to produce the best outcome for the least cost.

"Cost efficiency" is a term used to describe the concept of obtaining the best outcome for the least cost[6]. Cost efficiency cannot be determined without knowing both the cost and the result of care provided. Two protocols can be compared in terms of cost, but do they produce the same outcome? Likewise, two protocols may produce the same outcome, but are there differences in cost?

Outcome measures are not an end in themselves. Some interest in outcomes is generated because of external requirements from payers or their potential as a marketing tool. But they are most useful in targeting quality-improvement activities and evaluating utilization and costs. Therefore, outcome measurement is the starting point in evaluating the effect of changes in care practices made in response to prospective payment. For example, with PPS, an agency may choose a strategy to decrease skilled-nursing visits for patients with congestive heart failure (CHF). A decline in outcome measures for CHF patients, as compared to the time period prior to the change in number of visits, should trigger a more thorough process evaluation to determine whether the decrease in visits is the likely cause of the poorer outcomes. Or an agency may evaluate two different clinical paths for patients with hip replacement, and analyze outcomes and cost to determine the most efficient pattern of care.

Unfortunately, outcome measurement does not come without a cost. The data required to adequately measure outcomes must be sufficiently precise and standardized. This means most home-care providers will need to make changes in assessment protocols and data-collection processes. Without precise measures, the data are not sufficiently reliable. And without standardization, it is impossible to compare results among providers. Also, risk adjustment is necessary to account for the differences in the likelihood of patients achieving a positive outcome. Unadjusted outcome measures may indicate that an agency has poorer outcomes than the average; however, that difference may be related to the agency's having a patient population with more severe problems and less expectation to improve. In the end, the burden of data collection must be weighed against the value of having adequate information to direct changes in care practices and the costs of providing care.

Information is the basis for power. In the case of a PPS, those organizations that are skillful in identifying, compiling, and analyzing their data are most likely to be successful in the changing environment. Home-care organizations must integrate financial and clinical information. They will be challenged to manage more data than they have in the past in order to thrive in the era of cost containment and accountability for quality.

References
1. HCFA, *The Home Health Agency Prospective Payment Demonstration, Phase II* (Cambridge, MA: Abt Associates, Inc., 1994).
2. Code of Federal Regulations, Part 42, Public Health, Section 409.45 Dependent services requirements (Washington, DC: U.S. Government Printing Office, 1995).
3. HCFA, unpublished information, "Home Health Utilization Groups" (HHUG's #2) (1994).
4. HCFA, Request for Proposal (RFP # 96-013/PK), "Case-Mix Adjustment for a National Home Health Prospective Payment System" (1996).
5. Center for Health Policy Studies, "Understanding and Choosing Clinical Performance Measures for Quality Improvement: Development of a Typology" (Agency for Health Care Policy and Research PB95-184784) (Springfield, VA: National Technical Information Service, 1995).

6. L. Scott, "Looking Beyond Cost," *Modern Health Care* (February 28, 1994): 36–40.

APPENDIX A

Revised Unified Proposal for a
Prospective Payment System for Medicare Home Health Services
March 28, 1996

Developed jointly by
The National Association for Home Care (NAHC)
and
The PPS Work Group

This plan is a modification of the original unified plan submitted to Congress in 1995 as an alternative to Congressional movement to impose co-pays on Medicare home-care services or to bundle home-care payments into payments to hospitals. The modifications were made to the original proposal to respond to concerns about implementation feasibility raised by HCFA.

This plan incorporates the best elements of the 1995 home-care PPS provisions in HR 2491 passed by Congress and HR 2530. It represents months of work and refinement by the home-care industry. The plan calls for a three-phase approach to achieving episodic PPS. It starts with an interim PPS plan that utilizes existing data and processes and moves to an episodic PPS with a refined case-mix adjustor.

PPS is a more efficient, cost-effective alternative for achieving reductions in the growth of expenditures than co-pays or bundling of home-care services. PPS can accomplish this goal without jeopardizing beneficiary health and safety, or increasing out-of-pocket costs.

APPENDIX B

Home Care's Plan to Implement Prospective Payment for
Medicare Home-health Services

I. Home Care's Goal

The goal of the home-care provider community is to manage the growth of Medicare home-health expenditures in a manner that promotes efficiency and preserves access to quality care for Medicare beneficiaries. This will be accomplished through the development and implementation of an episodic prospective payment system as soon as feasible. PPS is a more efficient, cost-effective

Prospective Payment **117**

alternative for achieving reductions in the growth of expenditures than co-pays or bundling of home-care services. PPS can accomplish this goal without jeopardizing beneficiary health and safety.

PPS will be phased in over time, culminating in an episodic prospective payment system plan that should
- be developed cooperatively by HHS, the industry, and Congress;
- be acceptable to the industry;
- include extended care;
- be submitted to Congress one year in advance of implementation, and within four years of enactment of legislation;
- be approved by Congress;
- include adjustments for new requirements (such as OSHA) or changes in technology or care practices; and
- be based on a case-mix adjustor that reflects the differences in cost for different types of patients.

II. An Interim PPS Plan

An interim PPS plan incorporating certain elements of the Congressional and Democratic proposals (HR 2491 and HR 2530) should be implemented commencing within six months of enactment and continue until it can be converted to a pure episodic prospective payment system (Phase III). The interim PPS plan should be based on the industry's design and set forth in legislative language. The interim plan is implemented in phases to provide HCFA sufficient time to collect necessary data and to develop required processes and procedures. Current coverage criteria for Medicare home-health services should be maintained and no coverage shifted to Part B.

III. Time Line for PPS Phase-In

Enact Legislation	Begin Data Collection	Begin Phase I Interim PPS	Begin Phase II Interim PPS	Report to Congress on Episodic PPS	Expected Implementation Phase III Episodic PPS
0	2 mo.	6 mo.	24—30 mo.	48 mo.	60 mo.

IV. PPS Specifications

A. Data Collection

HCFA is mandated to begin immediately to develop a database upon which a fair and accurate case-mix adjustor can be developed and implemented. The database must be able to link case-mix data with cost (and utilization) data.

The database must include a sample sufficiently large to support the development of statistically valid estimates of payment rates and limits for the geographic area used (e.g., MSA/non-MSA, national, census region).

The database must contain at least

- items for the 18-category Phase II case-mix adjustor;
- HCFA form 485;
- UB-92; and
- additional data items that may contribute to a more accurate case-mix system, developed with industry participation (such as items from OASIS).

Payment rates and limits shall be adjusted to reflect cost of data collection.

Effective date: 60 days after enactment

B. *Phase-In of PPS Beginning With the Interim Plan*
   Phase I
   Prospectively set standard per-visit payment (as in HR 2491) with an annual aggregate per-patient limit that applies to all visits (as in HR 2530)
   Effective date: 6 months after enactment
   All currently allowable costs related to nonroutine medical supplies will be included in the database for calculating the per-visit rate, per-visit limit, and aggregate limits.

   Per-visit payment
   - standard per visit rate for each discipline calculated (as in HR 2491) as follows
     the national average amount paid per visit under Medicare to home-health agencies for each discipline during the most recent 12-month cost reporting period ending on or before 12-31-94 and updated by the home-health market-basket index, except that the labor-related portion of such rate shall be adjusted by the area wage index applicable under section 1886(d)(3)(E) for the area in which the agency is located
   - amounts in excess of the per visit rate, up to a limit as defined below, may be paid if
     1) an HHA can demonstrate costs above the payment rate; and
     2) quarterly reports demonstrate that total payments will not exceed the agency aggregate limit.
   - the payment rates and limits are calculated initially from the base-year costs and cost limits and updated by the home-health market-basket index to the date of implementation; they are updated annually by the market-basket index
   - base year for payment rates and cost limits—1994 (using settled cost reports)

Agency annual aggregate per-patient payment limit
- base year for aggregate payment limit—1995 utilization data for each agency
- the blended annual per-patient limit is based on the reasonable cost per unduplicated patient in the base year (1994 cost per visit updated, multiplied by 1995 utilization) and updated by the home-health market-basket index; calculation based 75% on agency data and 25% on census-region data for 12 months following implementation of Phase I, then 50% agency data and 50% census-region data
- the blended annual aggregate per-patient limit is equal to the number of unduplicated patients served in the year multiplied by the per-patient blended limit
- census region: the nine census-region geographic areas (New England, Middle Atlantic, East North Central, West North Central, South Atlantic, East South Central, West South Central, Mountain, Pacific)

Sharing savings
HHAs that are able to keep their total payments for the year below their annual aggregate per-patient cap and below 125% of the census-region cost/utilization experience shall receive a payment equal to 50% of the difference between the total per-visit payments and the agency's aggregate limit. Such payments may not exceed 10% of an agency's aggregate Medicare per-visit payments in a year.

Phase I in place 18 months (no longer than 24 months)

Phase II
Prospectively set standard per-visit payment with an annual aggregate episode limit for days 1–120 (as in HR 2491); and an annual aggregate per-patient limit for visits after 120 days
- continue per-visit payment as in Phase I
- an episode is 120 days; post-120-day care is paid per visit with an annual aggregate per-patient blended limit for the post-120-day period that is separate from the 1—120-day annual aggregate episode limit
- the HHA is credited for a new episode limit if there is a period of 45 days without Medicare-covered home health-care services following the 120-day episode (if a patient is readmitted before a new episode can be started, the agency is paid per visit subject to the aggregate episode limit if within the first 120 days, or the separate post-120-day aggregate per-patient blended limit if   after 120 days)
- the 18-category Phase II case-mix adjustor is applied to the first 120 days, or a more accurate one if available
- the per-episode limit (as in HR 2491) is equal to the mean number of visits for each discipline during the 120-day episode of a case-mix cat-

egory in an area during the base year multiplied by the per-visit payment rate for each discipline
- the annual aggregate episode limit (as in HR 2491) is equal to the number of episodes of each case-mix category during the fiscal year multiplied by the per episode limit determined for such case-mix category for such fiscal year
- the region for the episode limit—MSA/non-MSA area
- the annual post-120-day per-patient blended limit is based on the reasonable cost per unduplicated patient receiving care beyond 120 days in the base year (1994 cost per visit updated, multiplied by 1995 utilization) and updated by the home-health market-basket index; calculation based 50% on agency data and 50% on census-region data
- the annual aggregate post-120-day per-patient blended limit is equal to the number of unduplicated patients receiving care beyond 120 days in the year multiplied by the per-patient blended limit
- the current certification and coverage guidelines continue

Sharing savings

HAS that are able to keep their total payments for the year below their annual aggregate episode and post-120-day per-patient caps; and the post-120-day per-patient payments below 125% of the census-region cost/utilization experience, shall receive a payment equal to 50% of the difference between the total per-visit payments and the agency's aggregate limits. Such payments may not exceed 10% of an agency's aggregate Medicare per-visit payments in a year.

Phase III (as noted under the goal in section I)
Per-episode PPS
- developed cooperatively by HAS, the industry, and Congress
- acceptable to the industry
- includes extended care
- must be submitted to Congress one year in advance of implementation and within four years of enactment of legislation
- approved by Congress
- adjustments for new requirements (such as OSHA) or changes in technology or care practices
- case-mix adjustor that reflects the differences in cost for different types of patients

C. Additional Specifications That Apply to All Phases

1. *Exceptions*: The Secretary shall provide for an exemption from, or an exception and adjustment to, the methods for determining payment limits where extraordinary circumstances beyond the home-health agency's control

includingoutliers and the case mix of such home-health agency, create unintended distortions in care requirements not accounted for in the case-mix adjustor payment system. The Secretary shall develop a method for monitoring expenditures for such exceptions. Methods should be developed to allow for additional home-care expenditures when they are found to decrease total Medicare expenditures.

2. *Quality*: Any prospective payment system must ensure that home-health agencies do not seek to become more cost effective by sacrificing quality. The Secretary will ensure that the quality of services remains high by implementing a revised survey and certification process which emphasizes patient satisfaction and successful outcomes.

Home-health agencies will be required to provide covered services to beneficiaries to the extent that those services are determined by the beneficiary's physician to be medically necessary.

There will be established a means for beneficiary due process to challenge care and coverage determinations first through internal provider grievance procedures, then through external PRO review.

There will be established a mechanism for quality review for instances of significant variation in utilization by providers (this can address both visits and admissions).

About the Author

Karen Pace, MAN, RN, is Vice President for Research, Regulatory Affairs, and Education at the National Association for Home Care (NH). She was actively involved in the development and analysis of the industry's Unified Proposal for a Prospective Payment System for Medicare Home-Health Services. Pace is involved in reviewing and disseminating information on HCFA's plans to implement outcome-based quality-improvement requirements for Medicare-certified home-health agencies.

Pace has an MS in nursing. She has a wide variety of home-care experience including home health, hospice, and home infusion therapy. She has functioned in clinical, management, and educational roles.